Comprehensive Guide to Education in Anesthesia

Elizabeth A.M. Frost
Editor

Comprehensive Guide to Education in Anesthesia

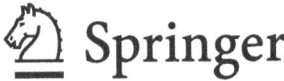

Editor
Elizabeth A.M. Frost
Department of Anesthesiology
Icahn Medical Center at Mount Sinai
New York, NY, USA

ISBN 978-1-4614-8953-5   ISBN 978-1-4614-8954-2 (eBook)
DOI 10.1007/978-1-4614-8954-2
Springer New York Heidelberg Dordrecht London

Library of Congress Control Number: 2013953289

© Springer Science+Business Media New York 2014
This work is subject to copyright. All rights are reserved by the Publisher, whether the whole or part of the material is concerned, specifically the rights of translation, reprinting, reuse of illustrations, recitation, broadcasting, reproduction on microfilms or in any other physical way, and transmission or information storage and retrieval, electronic adaptation, computer software, or by similar or dissimilar methodology now known or hereafter developed. Exempted from this legal reservation are brief excerpts in connection with reviews or scholarly analysis or material supplied specifically for the purpose of being entered and executed on a computer system, for exclusive use by the purchaser of the work. Duplication of this publication or parts thereof is permitted only under the provisions of the Copyright Law of the Publisher's location, in its current version, and permission for use must always be obtained from Springer. Permissions for use may be obtained through RightsLink at the Copyright Clearance Center. Violations are liable to prosecution under the respective Copyright Law.

The use of general descriptive names, registered names, trademarks, service marks, etc. in this publication does not imply, even in the absence of a specific statement, that such names are exempt from the relevant protective laws and regulations and therefore free for general use.

While the advice and information in this book are believed to be true and accurate at the date of publication, neither the authors nor the editors nor the publisher can accept any legal responsibility for any errors or omissions that may be made. The publisher makes no warranty, express or implied, with respect to the material contained herein.

Printed on acid-free paper

Springer is part of Springer Science+Business Media (www.springer.com)

*To my sister and friend,
Dr. Jean Margaret Handscombe, an educator*

Foreword

Having recently completed my tenth board certification/recertifcation examination over the past 20 years, I have a few important thoughts. First, the education process and the manner in which we measure knowledge and competence in all fields, including in Anesthesiology and its subspecialties, are constantly changing. Who could have imagined tests on cadavers, computers, or simulators just a few years ago? Second, technology, medications, and procedures that were once considered small parts of our practice have evolved. Ultrasound, fluoroscopy-guided pain procedures, and transesophageal echocardiography are all very clear examples of changes which have significantly enhanced and changed the way we practice anesthesia in each of our specialty areas. Elaborate ultrasound-guided regional anesthesia techniques in all patient populations, transesophageal real-time views of the heart in cardiovascular surgery, and TAP blocks in obstetric anesthesia patients are improvements over how we practiced anesthesia just a few decades ago. Third, the development of electronic medical records and computer technology has dramatically changed our practices in all aspects. Fourth, newer boards and reconfigured tests have evolved. The American Board of Anesthesiology now offers is now an exam with three parts. Recertification sites for the American Board of Anesthesiology will now include simulation. In this regard, the last board examination that I recently completed, the relatively new American Board of Interventional Pain Physicians, having only been created a few years ago, involves four parts, a basic/clinic science portion, a substance abuse section, a coding and compliance section, and an oral/practical section. This is reflective of changes in our practices and within each anesthesia subspecialty.

This carefully constructed book by one of the great leaders in our field, Dr. Elizabeth A. M. Frost, M.D., provides an A–Z user-friendly text from leaders in our field to describe all aspects of education. From its historic evolution, the book touches in detail on all topics of relevant interest. Some of these include closed claims analysis, residency and fellowship training and requirements, the board certification process, the role of simulation, research, and community/global outreach and education. Medical students, health care professionals, and administrators may better understand the field of Anesthesiology after reading this book. Anesthesiologists at all levels will appreciate the many changes that have taken place in recent years. Dr. Frost, who has been a mentor to so many, including myself, has created a wonderful and important book for all to enjoy!

New Orleans, LA, USA   Alan David Kaye

Preface

After a less than satisfying stint as a surgeon (no cures, just cut it out), I spent some time in internal medicine. There I found that arguments were the norm... does the Lancet publish better studies than the New England Journal of Medicine or does the New England Journal of Medicine report more up to date data than the Lancet? This indecision was not for me. Still undaunted, I went on to obstetrics where I was appalled at women's inhumanity to women (come on, push... it doesn't hurt that much!). Well it does hurt that much. At about this time it occurred to me that people expected essentially two things from their doctor: deliver the baby and take away the pain. Having conquered (?) the first part, anesthesia seemed the only career for me. And so, 50 years ago I started on what is still for me an amazing learning experience. I had no idea that this specialty could hold so much. From open drop ether and cyclopropane with a finger on the pulse as our only check that the patient was still alive to elaborate machines with a vast array of monitoring equipment, all the while caring for patients that may be so ill that their continued existence seems to hang by a thread, my education through these years has been monumental. And for that I have so many mentors to thank. From my first chair, Dr. Artusio, to my second appointment at the Albert Einstein College of Medicine with Drs. Orkin and Hershey, and later Dr. Goldiner, and now with Dr. Reich at Mount Sinai. I am grateful to all the educators who have helped others better understand the magic of anesthesia. And, of course, to all the contributors to the continuing education series in Anesthesiology News, now more than 30 years old and over 300 lessons long, thank you for making me continue to learn.

In the *Comprehensive Guide to Education in Anesthesia*, educators from many different aspects of anesthesia have all given their time and expertise to review current practice of learning in our specialty. My special thanks to them all.

Of course, as ever, extra thanks are due to the staff at Springer, to Shelley Reinhardt, Joanna Perey, and Kevin Wright, who have all worked hard to keep us on the right track.

New York, NY, USA   Elizabeth A.M. Frost

Contents

1   **Introduction and Historical Accounting** 1
    Elizabeth A.M. Frost

2   **Teaching by Example: Best Practices for Education in the Operating Room and the Lecture Hall** 15
    Ethan O. Bryson

3   **Learning from Incident Reporting and Closed Claims Analyses** 27
    Julia Metzner, Karen L. Posner, and Karen B. Domino

4   **Residency Training** 41
    Daniel Katz and Alan Sim

5   **Requirements for a Fellowship** 59
    Sarah AbdelFattah and William Peruzzi

6   **Teaching Clinical Science to Medical Students** 69
    Chanannait Paisansathan and Verna L. Baughman

7   **Mentorship in Anesthesia** 87
    Monica S. Vavilala and Elizabeth A.M. Frost

8   **The Process of Board Certification** 99
    Ann E. Harman and Cynthia A. Lien

9   **Maintenance of Certification in Anesthesiology Program** 117
    Natalie F. Holt

10   **Evaluation of Anesthesiology Residents** 129
    John E. Tetzlaff

11   **Giving Feedback to Superiors-Attending Evaluation** 147
    Shara Steiner Brody, Julie Oppenheimer, and Michael C. Lewis

12	**The Place for Simulation Teaching**...	159
	Judy G. Johnson	
13	**The Role of Continuing Medical Education**	173
	Christina L. Jeng and Francine S. Yudkowitz	
14	**Multidisciplinary Teaching: The Interaction of the Specialties**..........	183
	Michael Yarborough, Brian McClure, and Santiago Gomez	
15	**Research in Education**...	195
	Robert Fallar, Reena Karani, and Erica Friedman	
16	**The Place of Global Education in Anesthesia**..	205
	Angela Enright	
17	**Community Outreach**..	215
	Jordan Brand and Clifford Gevirtz	
18	**Substance Abuse Recognition and Prevention Through Education**	229
	Ethan O. Bryson	
Index..		243

Contributors

Sarah AbdelFattah, M.D. Department of Anesthesiology, Perioperative Medicine & Pain Management, Jackson Memorial Hospital, University of Miami Miller School of Medicine, Miami, FL, USA

Verna L. Baughman, M.D. Department of Anesthesiology, University of Illinois at Chicago, Chicago, IL, USA

Jordan Brand, M.D. Department of Anesthesiology, San Francisco VA Medical Center, University of California, San Francisco, CA, USA

Shara Steiner Brody, D.O. Department of Health Informatics, University of Miami Miller School of Medicine, Plantation, FL, USA

Ethan O. Bryson, M.D. Department of Anesthesiology and Psychiatry, The Icahn School of Medicine at Mount Sinai, New York, NY, USA

Karen B. Domino, M.D., M.P.H. Department of Anesthesiology and Pain Medicine, University of Washington, Seattle, WA, USA

Angela Enright University of British Columbia, Royal Jubilee Hospital, Victoria, BC, Canada

Robert Fallar, M.S. The Mount Sinai Medical Center, New York, NY, USA

Department of Medicine, Icahn School of Medicine at Mount Sinai, New York, NY, USA

Erica Friedman, M.D., F.A.C.P. Sophie Davis School of Biomedical Education, City College, City University of New York, New York, NY, USA

Elizabeth A.M. Frost, M.D. Icahn Medical Center at Mount Sinai, New York, NY, USA

Clifford Gevirtz, M.D., M.P.H. LSU Health Sciences Center, New Orleans, LA, USA

Santiago Gomez, M.D. Department of Anesthesiology, Tulane School of Medicine, New Orleans, LA, USA

Ann E. Harman, Ph.D. The American Board of Anesthesiology, Inc., Raleigh, NC, USA

Natalie F. Holt, M.D., M.P.H. Department of Anesthesiology, Yale University School of Medicine, New Haven, CT, USA

Department of Anesthesiology, VA Connecticut Healthcare System, West Haven Campus, West Haven, CT, USA

Christina L. Jeng, M.D. Department of Anesthesiology, Icahn School of Medicine at Mount Sinai, New York, NY, USA

Judy G. Johnson, M.D. Department of Anesthesiology, School of Medicine, Louisiana State University Health Sciences Center, New Orleans, LA, USA

Reena Karani, M.D., M.H.P.E. Department of Medical Education, Icahn School of Medicine at Mount Sinai, New York, NY, USA

Daniel Katz, M.D. Department of Anesthesiology, Icahn School of Medicine at Mount Sinai, New York, NY, USA

Michael C. Lewis, M.D. University of Florida College of Medicine Jacksonville, Jacksonville, FL, USA

Cynthia A. Lien, M.D. Department of Anesthesiology, New York Presbyterian Hospital, Weill Cornell Medical College, New York, NY, USA

Brian McClure, M.D. Department of Anesthesiology, Tulane School of Medicine, New Orleans, LA, USA

Julia Metzner, M.D. Department of Anesthesiology and Pain Medicine, University of Washington, Seattle, WA, USA

Julia Metzner, M.D. Department of Anesthesiology and Pain Medicine, University of Washington, Seattle, WA, USA

Julie Oppenheimer, M.D. Department of Anesthesiology, University of Miami Miller School of Medicine, Plantation, FL, USA

Chanannait Paisansathan, M.D. Department of Anesthesiology, University of Illinois at Chicago, Chicago, IL, USA

William Peruzzi, M.D., S.M., F.C.C.M. Department of Anesthesiology, Perioperative Medicine & Pain Management, Jackson Memorial Hospital, University of Miami Miller School of Medicine, Miami, FL, USA

Karen L. Posner, Ph.D. Department of Anesthesiology and Pain Medicine, University of Washington, Seattle, WA, USA

Alan Sim, M.D. Department of Anesthesiology, Icahn School of Medicine at Mount Sinai, New York, NY, USA

Contributors

John E. Tetzlaff, M.D. Cleveland Clinic Lerner College of Medicine, Case Western Reserve University, Cleveland, OH, USA

Department of General Anesthesia, Anesthesiology Institute, Cleveland Clinic, Cleveland, OH, USA

Monica S. Vavilala, M.D. Department of Anesthesiology & Pain Medicine, University of Washington, Seattle, WA, USA

Michael Yarborough, M.D. Department of Anesthesiology, Tulane School of Medicine, New Orleans, LA, USA

Francine S. Yudkowitz, M.D., F.A.A.P. Department of Anesthesiology, Icahn School of Medicine at Mount Sinai, New York, NY, USA

Chapter 1
Introduction and Historical Accounting

Elizabeth A.M. Frost

"Anesthesia," from the Greek αν-, *an-*, "without"; and αἴσθησις, *aisthēsis*, "sensation" Attributed in 1846 by Oliver Wendell Holmes, Sr.

"Education" from the Latin *ēducātiō* (a bringing up) from *ēdūcō* (I train, I lead out)

"To educate," from the Latin educatus, (re*ar*, educate), coined 1447 ("education" meaning to provide schooling first expressed in 1588 by Shakespeare)

Early Times

Attempts have been made since the earliest times to alleviate pain and suffering [1]. The use of natural substances as soporifics such as alcohol, herbs, including mandrake, henbane, cannabis and opium and the saliva from the chewing of coca leaves in Peru has been well documented for centuries [2, 3]. Two eminent Chinese surgeons, Pien Ch'iao and Hua T'O, in the first and second century AD were said to be so skilled in the use of anesthesia that they were able to operate painlessly [4]. The German sinologist Dr. Erich Hauer believed that the "bubbling drug medicine" that they used was opium, probably dissolved in wine. Pedanius Dioscorides (40–90 CE) a Greek surgeon in the army of Nero described the use of many herbs, especially opium. His work, *De Materia Medica*, was the standard pharmacopeia for some 1,500 years, and in it he noted "sleeping potions such as opium or mandragora are applied to such people as shall be cut or cauterized…for they do not apprehend pain because they are overcome with dead sleep…but used too much they make men speechless (i.e., dead)." He wrote of wine made from the mandrake that could induce anesthesia, defined as the sense of an absence of sensation in patients about to undergo surgery [5]. Also the Greek word, Karoun, from which carotid is derived,

E.A.M. Frost, M.D. (✉)
Icahn Medical Center at Mount Sinai, 1 Gustav L Levy Place, KCC 8-46, Box 1010, New York, NY, USA
e-mail: elzfrost@aol.com

means to fall asleep and he may have recognized that pressure on the carotid artery causes loss of consciousness. Of note, Dioscorides' use of the word "anesthesia" anticipated Holmes recommendation to Morton by almost 1,800 years.

In the seventh century Paulus Aeginata in perhaps what is the biggest act of plagiarism ever committed in the medical world collected all the works of Hippocrates, Galen, Dioscorides, and Areteus, among others, and produced seven books, the last of which is over 600 pages long and is devoted to herbal remedies, especially to the pain-alleviating powers of opium [6].

A "soporific sponge" ("sleep sponge") was introduced by the Salerno School of Medicine in the late twelfth century, although there is some evidence that it may have been offered to Christ on the cross (Matthew 27:48, Mark 15:36, John 19:29). The sponge was soaked in a dissolved solution of opium, mandragora, hemlock juice, and other substances. It was then dried and stored until just before surgery when it was moistened and held against the patient's face. When all went well, it worked [7].

No doubt the recipes for the treatment of all ills and the relief from pain were handed down, often from mothers to daughters and the therapies often kept as well-guarded secrets, but orally ingested substances were not reliable in the amount of pain relief they could effect. Inhalation agents were needed.

Anesthesia for Entertainment

Ether was first made by a Spanish physician Raymond Lullus in 1275. He did not use it on humans and neither did Paracelsus in the sixteenth century; the latter simply anesthetized chickens [8]. Frobenius named the substance "ether" in 1730, a Greek word for heavenly [8]. Nitrous oxide which was considered lethal even in small doses was discovered by Priestley in 1772. However, Davy experimented on himself in 1799 and found the gas made him laugh. Thus the beginnings of anesthesia as we know it started with the use of inhaled gases for recreation and shows. Humphrey Davy at the Pneumatic Institute administered his laughing gas to many luminaries of the time including the poets Southey and Coleridge, Roget (of thesaurus fame), James Watt (the engineer), and Wedgewood (the potter), among many others [9]. But, although Davy had written (at the age of 21) a 580-page summary of the actions of N_2O, he did not appreciate the gas as a part of pain relief and he soon went on to other pursuits (gun powder being one of them) [10]. It was to fall to an American, Crawford Long, to recognize the anesthetic effects of ether, perhaps when he used it during ether frolics at the University of Pennsylvania. He anesthetized a student, James Venable on March 30, 1842, for removal of a tumor on his neck. The operation was not announced until 1849 [11].

By 1819, Stockman and Phineas Taylor Barnum, both from New York, were among several other itinerant "professors" of chemistry who recognized the entertainment and financial prospects of nitrous oxide [12, 13]. These showmen traveled throughout the United States lecturing on gases and demonstrating the exhilarating effects of nitrous oxide and ether. Barnum at that time was the proprietor of the American Museum in New York, advertised as "a place of education, edification, and amusement." He arranged with another "professor of chemistry," Gardner Colton, to organize many demonstrations of the enjoyable effects of nitrous oxide [14]. At one of these shows, Horace Wells appreciated the anesthetic effects of the inhalation of the gas. Although his public demonstration of the anesthetic effects of nitrous oxide failed, his sometime friend, Morton, achieved success with ether on October 30, 1846.

Discovered in 1831, chloroform was also used first as an "after dinner entertainment" by James Young Simpson in Edinburgh in November 1847. When his guests quickly fell asleep, Simpson, an obstetrician, recognized the potential use in his practice. One week later, he reported on 30 painless deliveries to the Edinburgh Medico-Chirurgical Society [15]. John Snow, perhaps the first physician anesthetist, in London quickly adopted use of the agent.

Anesthetic Practice in the Nineteenth Century

Unlike surgery where "schools" of medicine and associations of philosophers, priest-physicians, and practitioners had been established for centuries throughout Greece (the Hippocratic schools of Knidan and Koan were only two) and all over the Arab world and Europe, there does not appear to have been formal classes in administration of anesthesia before the end of the nineteenth century. Although one could apprentice to general surgeons, urologists, and obstetricians, among many others, administration of pain-killing measures was considered a task for just about anyone.

Unfortunately, chloroform is not as safe an agent as ether, especially when administered by an untrained practitioner (medical students, nurses, and occasionally members of the public were often pressed into giving anesthetics or the surgeon both administered the anesthetic and performed the surgery). These practices led to many deaths from the use of chloroform that (with hindsight) might have been preventable. The first fatality directly attributed to chloroform anesthesia was recorded on January 28, 1848, after the death of Hannah Greener, a healthy 15-year-old who underwent removal of a toenail [16]. The anesthetic was administered by a surgeon, Mr. Meggison, while his assistant, Mr. Lloyd, removed the nail. Ms. Greener died within 3 min. Both Snow and Simpson quickly became involved in the controversy surrounding the death of the girl. Simpson maintained that her death was unrelated to the gas but rather due to the brandy and water given to her in an attempt to revive her [17]. Snow, on the other hand, wrote that "the fatal result should be attributed to the action of the chloroform on the nervous centers having extended so far as to put a stop to respiration" [18]. In other words, chloroform was more potent than ether and a fatal depth could be reached much faster. The physician administering the anesthetic had no monitors other than his finger on the pulse and his visual inspection of the patient. He also had little knowledge about the pharmacology of the anesthetic nor of effective methods or drugs for resuscitation. He had no access to experts and most of all he had had no training in anesthesia. The medical community began to realize that anesthesia could be a mixed blessing and was not as safe as had been suggested. Some education was essential.

An opportunity for education might have been possible about this time. In May 1845, a group of orthodox physicians met in New York City to hold a national convention. They reconvened 2 years later at the Academy of National Sciences in Philadelphia. Under the leadership of Nathan Davis, the American Medical Association was founded. A committee on medical education was appointed and a few years later a standing committee on surgery came into being. Forty-eight pages were devoted to anesthetic agents and management in the manual, but no formal training was recommended.

Appreciation of the Dangers of Anesthesia

Shortly after Greener's death, Snow published articles from May 1848 onwards "On Narcotism by the Inhalation of Vapours" in the London Medical Gazette, and by 1858 he reported on a series of the first 50 deaths from chloroform which are also detailed in a textbook (more than 150 pages of the 525 book are devoted to the causes and prevention of death) [19]. He was also involved with the production of equipment needed for the safer administration of inhalational anesthetics.

In France, Claude Bernard was appointed chair of medicine at the Collège de France after the death of Magendie in 1855. He gave a course of lectures there starting around 1869 on anesthetics and asphyxia. These lectures were edited from listeners' notes with additional new experiments by Bernard and published in book form in 1875. Why the famous physiologist gave a course in anesthetics is uncertain as he was a nonclinician and probably never anesthetized a human being. He considered anesthetics poisons noting that "poisons are veritable reagents of life, extremely delicate instruments which dissect vital units. I believe I am the first to consider the study of poisons from this point of view, and, in my opinion, studious attention to agents which modify the histological elements should form the common foundation of general physiology, pathology and therapeutics" [20].

By the latter half of the nineteenth century, surgeons began to appreciate that they alone or with an untrained assistant could not perform both surgery and anesthesia. In the United Kingdom, by 1860, Joseph Lister, of antisepsis fame and the professor of surgery at the Glasgow Royal Infirmary, was opposed to both specialist anesthetists and anesthetic apparatus, claiming that his clerks were superior to other trained chloroformists [21]. In fact he went as far as to say that the appointment of a special administrator of chloroform to a hospital not only was unnecessary but also had "the disadvantage of investing the administration of chloroform with an air of needless mystery" [22]. Idiosyncratic death due to chloroform was so rare that it could be left out of consideration. Shortly after Lister left Glasgow, one of his former students William Macewen was appointed surgeon in charge of wards at the same institution in 1869 with a very different attitude [23]. This (neuro)surgeon had developed an interest in laryngeal obstruction while he was at the fever hospital where there were many cases of diphtheria. He had developed a series of tubes that could be passed orally. He later adapted the technique of endotracheal intubation for surgery [24]. Macewen emphasized the importance of the anesthetic and the solemn responsibility of the administrator. He insisted on medical student training and only those who had achieved a certificate of proficiency after successfully completing a written examination and practical test of 12 chloroform anesthetics could care for his patients. "Sir William was very particular indeed about anaesthetics and each student on his firm received a carefully designed course of several weeks supervised training on the administration, especially of chloroform…and this together with the practical instruction, gave a through grounding in anesthesia as we knew it at the time" [25]. However, although all medical students at Glasgow University in 1880 were required to have a certificate of proficiency in vaccination, only those who were assigned to Macewen's wards had anesthetic training. Macewen persisted, and on October 9, 1882, Mr. McEwan, chairman of the board of the Royal Infirmary, proposed that the pathologist should deliver a course of lectures on anesthetics at the beginning of the winter session and a certificate should be awarded. The resolutions were amended by the omission of "pathologist" in November and approved by the medical staff a few weeks later [26]. Unfortunately, early in 1883, a "resident" (a rather loose term for someone who lived in the hospital) administered chloroform to an elderly patient who died intraoperatively. Mr. McEwan publicized the case in the local newspaper, the Glasgow Herald, stating that under no circumstances should untrained residents be permitted to administer chloroform. Two surgeons, Mr. James Morton and Dr. Leishman, responded immediately that anesthetics had been safely administered by many untrained individuals and surgeons should not be hampered by petty rules and regulations, requiring additional paper work. The bitter debate continued for several weeks in the newspaper but positive action was achieved. A special committee of the managers of the infirmary was formed on March 1, 1883, under the leadership of Professor WT Gairdner, who would become the president of the British Medical Association in 1888, to assess the level of education and regulations regarding the administration of anesthetics. A questionnaire was sent to medical superintendents of 40 hospitals and medical schools in the United Kingdom. The response rate was just under 50 % (Table 1.1).

Of the four hospitals that had specialist anesthetists, three were in London and the fourth in Aberdeen. Fatalities were related to the patient's poor condition rather than to the anesthetic. After tabulation of the results, several changes were incorporated at the Glasgow Royal Infirmary by March 7, 1883, including mandatory instruction in anesthesia with practical demonstration of competence. Only those who had completed the course and obtained a certificate were allowed to give anesthesia, except in dire emergencies. House officers were not to operate or administer anesthesia unsupervised. An operating log was to be completed after every operation, and anesthetic deaths had to be reported and investigated. These modifications were in place by 1884 [27].

Table 1.1 Survey sent to all hospitals in the United Kingdom regarding anesthesia education and training in 1883

Questions	Yes	No
Are there formal regulations?	8	10
Is special instruction provided?	9	9
Are resident clerks permitted to work unsupervised?	16	2
Are resident anesthetic assistants or principal officers allowed to give anesthesia?	9 Assistants 3 Principal officers 4 Allowed both	
Are residents qualified to practice medicine and was anesthesia training required?	16	2 6 No requirement for training
Is there a specialist for administration of anesthetics?	4	11
Have fatal accidents occurred?	13	3
Was practice modified by accidents?	0	18

Beginnings of Education in Anesthesia

Although anesthetic training was firmly established in Glasgow, the struggle remained in the rest of the United Kingdom. The London Society of Anaesthetists was established in 1893 (it was to form the Anaesthetic section of the Royal Society of Medicine in 1908), but considerable resistance remained to mandating of training in anesthesia. That anesthesia was well established in surgical practice is undisputed. As reported in the *Boston Medical and Surgical Journal* (after 1928, the *New England Journal of Medicine*) in 1888, on the advances during the reign of Queen Victoria, the discovery and incorporation of anesthesia (along with antisepsis) was "epoch" making and "each has done as much for surgery as the discovery of hemostatics and when combined may, I think, be said to excel even steam and electricity in their gracious benefits to mankind" (Sir George MacLeod) [27]. "The lion heart is no more necessary for surgery!" [28] Change still came slowly. No doubt it was mainly through the efforts of Hewitt that the General Medical Council determined in 1911 that all medical examining bodies must produce evidence of satisfactory instruction in anesthetic administration, a requirement that was not to be put in place in the United States for some 50 years [25]. Hewitt was the senior anesthetist and instructor at the London Hospital. Starting in 1898 he published many lectures, which he had delivered at the London Hospital, in the Lancet on anesthetic care [29–34]. One of his earlier lectures remarked on the administration of 6,657 anesthetics in 1887 at the hospital. At the beginning of the lecture series, he noted that a system of recording anesthetics had been initiated at the hospital on January 1 [29]. He detailed the type of anesthesia given, the indications for the several mixtures, and the means of inhalation. Several combinations were used, including one which he labeled A.C.E. (1 part alcohol, 2 parts chloroform, and 3 parts ether). In a second lecture, he remarked on the 13 complications that had been encountered [30]. A few weeks later, yet another lecture focused on the three deaths (out of 6,657 administrations) that had occurred perioperatively and the after effects of anesthesia [31]. Dr. Hewitt blamed chloroform for only one of the deaths, the others being due to the poor condition of the patient or the stress of surgery. Later lectures dealt with recent developments in anesthetic administration (modifications to the Clover system and the Junker apparatus) [32]. He continued as a dedicated educator, publishing updated lectures in the Lancet for several years [33]. In a somewhat philosophical lecture in 1910, he noted that "Upon the continent where general anesthesia is not so fully developed as in this country, and where, as a result, accidents and unsatisfactory experiences are far more common, it is not surprising that intra-spinal and other methods of local anaesthetisation should obtain such a firm foothold. I cannot help thinking, too, that there are some surgeons who, being comparatively deficient in sensitiveness and accepting surgery and its various procedures as necessarily unpleasant, fail to realize the necessity of reducing or preventing as far a possible mental as well as all physical pain" [34].

Textbooks to Further Education

Before the turn of the century, several textbooks had appeared both in the United Kingdom and in the United States including *Artificial Anaesthesia and Anaesthetics* by HM Lyman (1881, William Wood, New York). Dr. Lyman was a professor of physiology and diseases of the nervous system at Rush Medical Center in Chicago. At the London Hospital, texts were offered by Hewitt and RJ Probyn-Williams. In reviewing one of Hewitt's book, Jacobs wrote, "this book is…one of the many indications that the study of the administration of anaesthetics is receiving at length more of the attention which it deserves as regards the instruction of students" [35]. Perhaps the best known, *Anaesthetics*, was by Dudley Wilmot Buxton, a consultant anesthetist at the University College Hospital. By 1920, this book was already in the sixth edition. But in keeping with the practice of little specialization, a surgeon at Cook County Hospital in Chicago offered a short, 185 page, manual, *General and Local Anesthetics*. In the preface to the second edition in 1901 he wrote: "The competent anesthetist is the surgeon's most valuable assistant. Conscious of this fact, I have endeavored to present in a concise form techniques of surgical, general and local anesthesia. The book would have been made more academic but it was intended for the hospital interne and for the general practitioner" [36]. Several surgical textbooks included chapters on anesthetic administration, emphasizing mainly the associated mortality (or lack thereof) and morbidity. An example of this is Chapter 29 in *Modern Surgery* by Da Costa, arguably the most prolific surgeon of the day. Mortality associated with chloroform was quoted at 1:3,162 patients and for ether was 1:16,302 [37].

Anesthetic Providers: T Drysdale Buchanan

Anesthesia was still given by just about anyone in the health care industry in the United States at the turn of the century. To many it was considered to be a menial task, poorly paid, and at the discretion and direction of the surgeon who obtained the patents and paid the anesthetic provider. In 1890, physicians changed roles daily from surgeon to internist to analgesist. At the age of 21, T Drysdale Buchanan had just graduated from the Flower Fifth Ave. Hospital in New York (the Homeopathic College) in 1897 [38]. He acted first as a house surgeon in the Metropolitan Post-Graduate School of Medicine and became well acquainted with horse-drawn ambulance driving (and chasing) as he rotated variously through several disciplines including outpatient internal medicine, dermatology, genitourinary surgery, and surgery. In 1900 he related: "I was a junior at the old Homeopathic College and at that time it was the practice to take on four seniors to do the anesthesia for the clinics. Naturally, I was anxious to be selected as one of the four who were to do the anesthesias for old Dr. Helmuth's clinic…I finally got hold of a junior surgeon and asked him if he would allow me to give an anesthetic and he said "yes, indeed, you bring me a case for surgery and I will let you give the anesthetic" So I did. And that was about the only instruction I had in anesthesia." Dr. Buchanan continued for 40 years and became the most respected anesthetist in New York, appointed as professor of anesthesia at the Homeopathic Hospital, Columbia University, and several other hospitals in New York where his responsibilities extended to teaching. Although he published several articles, he did not contribute a textbook. As a captain in the US Army, he organized the Army School of Anesthesia at General Hospital No 14, Fort Oglethorpe, GA, and later at army hospitals in New York and New Jersey. He was a founder, past president, and representative of the American Society of Anesthesiologists and held certificate number 1 of the American Board of Anesthesiology.

The Long Island Society and the American Society of Anesthesiologists

More organizations were underway in New York. In October 1905, Dr. Adolph Frederick Erdman who was initially a gynecologist gathered a group of nine area physicians who were practicing anesthesia as a medical specialty at Long Island College Hospital. They formed the Long Island Society of Anesthetists, whose purpose was to promote the art and science of anesthesia. Annual dues were set at US$1 [39].

Not all were physicians (Table 1.2). Dr. Sanders was elected president. Unfortunately, the records of the society were lost in a fire at his house in 1911.

That same year, 1911, interest in the society and its scientific endeavors had grown. On October 28, 1911, at the New York Academy of Medicine, located at 40 East 41st Street in Manhattan, the name of the society was changed to the New York Society of Anesthetists. Minutes of that meeting were recorded by the secretary,

1 Introduction and Historical Accounting

Table 1.2 The founding members of the Long Island Society of Anesthetists

- Adolph Frederick Erdmann 37 years Anes
- Robert Ormiston Brockway 35 years Neurology
- George Lamb Buist, Jr 33 years Int Med
- Arthur Hubert Longstreet 32 years Obstetrics
- Herman Franklin McChesney 30 years Surgery
- George Frank Sammis 21 years Med student
- Harold A. Sanders 26 years Anes
- Louis Stork 26 years Surgery
- George William Tong 27 years Anes

HA Sanders. Thirty-four physicians attended the educational meeting. A new constitution was instituted on February 7, 1912, and reiterated the precepts of its founders for "the advancement of the science and art of Anesthesia...." The first elected president was Dr. James T. Gwathmey, whose textbook *Anesthesia* was to become a major educational resource over the next several decades, being published first in 1914 with a second edition in 1924. The society soon acquired nationwide prominence as membership requests from other states were received. In 1917, the New York State Society of Anesthetists, acting on behalf of its members and especially with the insistence of Dr. Buchanan, contacted the federal government to offer the services of organized anesthesia for the war effort.

Although it was not until 1936 that the American Society of Anesthetists as an offshoot of the New York Society became a reality Dr. Gwathmey refers to it by name as an educational force in the preface to the first edition of his textbook in 1914 [40]. In that same preface he wrote: "Every large hospital should have as a regular member of its staff an attending anesthetist." That same year Frank McMechan persuaded the *American Journal of Surgery* to include supplements on anesthesia and analgesia on a quarterly basis. McMechan was also instrumental in founding the International Anesthesia Research Society and the first journal devoted to anesthesia in the United States, *Anesthesia and Analgesia*, in 1922 [41]. The first issue of Anesthesiology, the official journal of the American Society of Anesthetists (changed to Anesthesiologists in 1944, ASA), appeared in July 1940 [40].

Anesthesia Education and Medical Schools

A major goal of the new society was to make education in anesthesia an integral part of all medical schools. An editorial in the *Journal of Surgery* in 1936 offered a dismal view: "In medical education, the notion has prevailed that if anesthesia were taught, it could be presented by any lecturer, regardless of training and special scientific background. Its importance was minimized; its interest depreciated. Graduates in medicine who became specialists did so by self proclamation. Their education was obtained through experience and by the slow, dangerous process of trial and error" [42]. In 1935, the Committee on Education of the Society sent questionnaires to 87 medical schools in the United States and Canada. Of the 75 replies, 58 listed instruction by a physician, as a separate course by nurses or as part of surgery or pharmacology. Seven had no instruction [40]. The Board of Directors approved a resolution in 1936: "It is to the best interest of the medical public that departments of anesthesia…shall be in charge of physicians who shall have direct supervision of teaching of this subject to undergraduates and graduates." The resolution went on to say that the teachers should themselves have had training in anesthesia and be certified as specialists in anesthesia [43]. The following year, seven universities asked the Education Committee to recommend directors for their anesthesia departments. Ralph M. Waters who had established the first truly academic department of anesthesia was quick to respond, offering several of his alumni (Waters had joined the new medical school of the University of Wisconsin in 1927 at a time when instruction in anesthesia was nonexistent and the field was practiced by only a few self-taught men [44]). Four hospitals were approved for residency programs in 1937, 17 in 1938, and 49 in 1945.

The American Board of Anesthesiology

In the meantime, the American Board of Anesthesiology, Inc. (ABA) was established as an affiliate of the American Board of Surgery, Inc. on June 2, 1937, an affiliation that was approved by the Advisory Board for Medical Specialties and the Council on Medical Education of the American Medical Association in 1938. In 1941 the Advisory Board for Medical Specialties approved the establishment of the American Board of Anesthesiology, Inc. (ABA) as a separate entity. In 1985 the ABA offered a certificate in critical care and in 1991 American Board of Medical Specialties (ABMS), the ABMS permitted the ABA to issue certificates in pain management that would be valid for 10 years.

Annual Meetings: Emery Rovenstine

Perhaps the greatest impetus to increased education and residency programs came from the returning veterans of World War II. Surgeons realized that appropriate anesthetic care was essential to survival in critically wounded individuals. In particular, Emery Rovenstine, who had served on the Army Advisory Board and was responsible for an order to Army general hospitals that placed anesthesiologists in charge of operating rooms, soon organized weekly anesthesia teaching rounds at New York University that developed into the Post-Graduate Assembly of the New York State Society of Anesthesiologists, an annual gathering that continues to this day as one of the most prestigious anesthesia meetings worldwide. The first assembly held under the auspices of the American Society of Anesthesiologists (ASA) and the New York State Society was a 2-day affair held at the Hotel Pennsylvania in New York. The second gathering at the Hotel New Yorker in 1947 was also under the auspices of the ASA, but thereafter, the two societies held separate annual meetings.

The Latter Half of the Twentieth Century

Another questionnaire was circulated by the Subcommittee on Medical Schools in 1956. Twenty-five percent still had no clinical anesthesia teaching. Moreover, in medical schools with anesthesiology divisions, only 50 % had departmental status, the rest were part of surgery [39]. Despite an increase in residency programs to 217 with 1,150 physicians in training, the report of the president of the ASA in 1960 still expressed considerable disappointment at the lack of progress in medical education. There had been no appreciable advances in incorporating anesthesiology into medical school curricula. Rather the ASA had concentrated more on increasing membership at the expense of education [39]. Efforts were renewed to establish standards for education in medical schools with limited success. Movies and pamphlets were produced and distributed to some 32,000 high schools in the country. In-training examinations, introduced in 1975, helped to better define the specialty. Gradually over the next decade, divisions of anesthesia became departments. Subspecialty organization began to emerge. The ASA issued standards for care and practice guidelines and parameters. With adherence to new monitoring standards, anesthesia became safer and more respected.

Into the Twenty-First Century

Today exposure to anesthesia education is required in all medical schools. Very few divisions of anesthesia as part of surgery remain. Board qualification is required for positions in academic centers and for most positions in community settings. Certification received after 2000 is time limited to 10 years. The voluntary ABA certification program was phased out in 2009 with the administration of the recertification examination in December 2009. The Maintenance of Certification in Anesthesia (MOCA) is now the only voluntary recertification option for diplomates certified before 2000. Nemergut, in reflecting on a practice of anesthesia and a curriculum laid out by Pauel Flagg, a New York anesthetist, in 1926, emphasized again that "anesthesia is the practice of medicine and its safe practice must be built on a thorough understanding of pharmacology, medicine and surgery. It must also be built upon scholarly investigation into the basic sciences" [45, 46].

Conclusion

Although surgical anesthesia has been a part of our culture for over 160 years, education and acceptance of the discipline as a specialty has a relatively short history of only about 30 years. At this point we would seem to have achieved a firm footing, but without continued education and awareness, as history tells us, we could still slip backwards.

References

1. Keyes TE. The history of surgical anesthesia. New York: Schumans; 1945. p. 4–14.
2. Gaggard HW. Devils, drugs and doctors. New York: Blue Ribbon; 1929. p. 93–6.
3. Fairley HB. Anesthesia in the Inca empire. Rev Esp Anestesiol Reanim. 2007;54:556–62.
4. Veith I. The Yellow Emperor's classic of internal medicine. Berkeley: University of California Press; 1973. p. 3.
5. Nuland SB. The origins of anesthesia. Birmingham, AL: The Classics of Medicine Library, Division of Gryphon Editions; 1983. p. 9.
6. Adams F (trans). The seven books of Paulus Aeginata, vol. 3. London: The Sydenham Society; 1847. p. 279–83.
7. Keil G. Spongia somnifera. Medieval milestones on the way to general and local anesthesia. Anaesthesist. 1989;38(12):643–8.
8. Toski JA, Bacon DR, Calverley RK. The history of anesthesiology. In: Barash PG, Cullen BF, Stoelting RK, editors. Clinical anesthesia. 4th ed. Philadelphia: Lippincott Williams & Wilkins; 2001. p. 3. ISBN 978-0-7817-2268.
9. Buxton DW. Anaesthetics: their uses and administration. 6th ed. Philadelphia: Blakiston's Son and Co.; 1920. p. 9–11, 105–10.
10. Davy H. Researches, chemical and philosophical; chiefly concerning nitrous oxide or dephlogisticated nitrous oxide and its respiration. London: Biggs and Cottle for J. Johnson; 1800.
11. Long CW. An account of the first use of sulphuric ether by inhalation as an anesthetic in surgical operations. South Med Surg J. 1849;5:705–13.
12. Frost EAM. History of nitrous oxide. In: Eger EI, editor. Nitrous oxide/N_2O. New York: Elsevier; 1985. p. 10–1.
13. Keys TE. An epitome of the history of surgical anesthesia. Anaesthetist. 1954;3(6):273–83.
14. Raper HR. Man against pain. New York: Prentice Hall; 1945. p. 68–78.
15. Simpson JY. Superinduction of anaesthesia in natural and morbid parturition: with cases illustrative of the use and effects of chloroform in obstetric practice Read to the Medico-Chirurgical Society of Edinburgh December 1st 1847. Published in Anaesthesia on the employment of chloroform and ether. Philadelphia: Lindsay and Blakiston 1849; p. 93–109.
16. Knight P, Bacon DR. An unexplained death. Anesthesiology. 2002;96:1250–3.
17. Simpson JY. Remarks on the alleged cause of death from the action of chloroform. Lancet. 1848;1:175–6.
18. Snow J. Remarks on the fatal case of inhalation of chloroform including additional explanations from Dr Meggison. Lond Med Gazette, New Series. 1848;6:277–8.
19. Snow J. On chloroform and other anaesthetics. London: John Churchill; 1858. p. 100–262.
20. Bernard C. Lectures on anesthetics and asphyxia. Paris: J.B. Bailliere and Son; 1875. p. 9.
21. Watt OM. Glasgow anaesthetists 1846–1946. Clydebank: James Pender; 1962. p. 15–7.
22. Sykes WS. Essays on the first hundred years of anaesthesia. Park Ridge: Wood Library of Anesthesiology; 1982. p. 128.
23. Miller JD. William Macewen: a master of surgery. Va Med. 1979;106:363–8.
24. Macewen W. The introduction of tubes into the larynx though the mouth instead of performing tracheotomy or laryngotomy. Br Med J. 1880;2:122–4.
25. James CDT. Sir William Macewen and anaesthesia. Anaesthesia. 1974;29:743–53 (quoting Professor Thomas Nicol, private assistant to Macewen).
26. Frost EAM. The contributions of Sir William Macewen, a pioneer neurosurgeon, to an early quality assurance survey in anesthesia. J Neurosurg Anesthesiol. 1991;3(1):28–33.
27. Macewen W. Presidential introduction to a discussion on anaesthesia. Glasgow Med J. 1890;34:321.
28. The British Medical Association. Report. Boston Med Surg J. 1888;69(9):203–5.
29. Hewitt FW. 6657 administrations of anaesthetics conducted at the London hospital during the year 1897. Lancet. 1898;151:483–6.
30. Hewitt FW. 6657 administrations of anaesthetics conducted at the London hospital during the year 1897. Lancet. 1898;151:623–7.

31. Hewitt FW. 6657 administrations of anaesthetics conducted at the London hospital during the year 1897. Lancet. 1898;151:772–5.
32. Hewitt FW. Some recent developments in the administration of anaesthetics. Lancet. 1901;157:916–9.
33. Hewitt FW. Three clinical lectures on general surgical anaesthesia. Lancet. 1907;170:139–42.
34. Hewitt FM. The aesthetics of an anaesthetics. Lancet. 1910;169:623–6.
35. Jacobs E. Book Review Select methods in the administration of nitrous oxide and ether. Ann Surg. 1888;9(4):317–8.
36. Heineck AP. Preface in; General and local anesthetics. 2nd ed. Chicago: Engelhard and Co.; 1901. p. 3.
37. DaCosta JC. Modern surgery. 4th ed. In: Chapter 29. Anesthesia and anesthetics. 1903. p. 868–91. http://jdc.jefferson.edu/dacosta_modernsurgery/16. Accessed 8 May 2013.
38. Dearborn FM. Tom Buchanan 1876–1940. Reprinted from the Quarterly of Phi Alpha Gamma May 1940; 7 pages Available from the Wood Library Museum, ASAhq.org.
39. Betcher AM. Historical development of the American Society of Anesthesiologists, Inc. In: Volpitto PP, Vandam LD, editors. The genesis of contemporary American anesthesiology. Springfield: Charles Thomas; 1982. p. 185–211.
40. Gwathmey JT. Anesthesia. 1st ed. New York: MacMillan Co.; 1914. p. 10.
41. Craig DB, Martin JT. Anesthesia and analgesia; 75 years of publication. Anesth Analg. 1997;85:237–47.
42. Wright AM. Anesthesia in the medical schools. Am J Surg. 1936;34(3):407.
43. Collected papers and minutes of the Long Island, New York and American Society of Anesthetists (1905–1936). Vol. 1. Minutes of April 9th meeting. In the collection of the wood Library Museum, American Society of Anesthesiologists.
44. Bacon DR, Ament R. Ralph Waters and the beginnings of academic anesthesiology in the United States: the Wisconsin template. J Clin Anesth. 1995;7(6):534–43.
45. Flagg PJ. Undergraduate and postgraduate instruction in anesthesia: with some considerations of hospital anesthesia service. Anesth Analg. 1926;5:247–53.
46. Nemergut EC. Education in anesthesia: then and now. Anesth Analg. 2012;114(1):5–6.

Chapter 2
Teaching by Example: Best Practices for Education in the Operating Room and the Lecture Hall

Ethan O. Bryson

Introduction

During the summer between my high school graduation and the start of college, I had the pleasure of working as an "explainer" for the Exploratorium in San Francisco, a hands-on museum of "science, art, and human perception" opened by Frank Oppenheimer in the fall of 1969 and located in the Palace of Fine Arts, a relic of the 1915 Panama-Pacific World Exhibition and Fair. Born out of a desire to transform the way science was taught, the Exploratorium (Fig. 2.1) was designed as a giant classroom, but one without desks in neat rows facing a chalkboard with students politely listening to their teacher. This place was completely different, and the philosophy that Oppenheimer brought to education was nothing short of revolutionary. The museum's exhibits were designed to be interactive and visitors were encouraged to touch, push, pull, and think their way through them. It was not enough to have a set of self-service instructions. As an "explainer" my job was to spend each day on the floor, engaging visitors to the museum, answering questions, and "explaining" the exhibits.

I was a recent high school graduate; all of the explainers were either high school students or recent graduates, and none of us had any formal science background or education experience. Yet within a day or two of being hired, we were expected to learn the (basic) physics behind the exhibits at least well enough to explain them to anyone who passed by or enquired. It did not matter that we were teenagers and not graduate students or science professors. I soon discovered that every interaction with a visitor, whether a quick answer to a short question or a long discussion about why the sky is blue or how a rainbow is formed, was a learning experience.

E.O. Bryson, M.D. (✉)
Department of Anesthesiology and Psychiatry, The Icahn School of Medicine at Mount Sinai, 1 Gustave L. Levy Plave, Box 1010, New York, NY, USA
e-mail: ethan.bryson@mountsinai.org

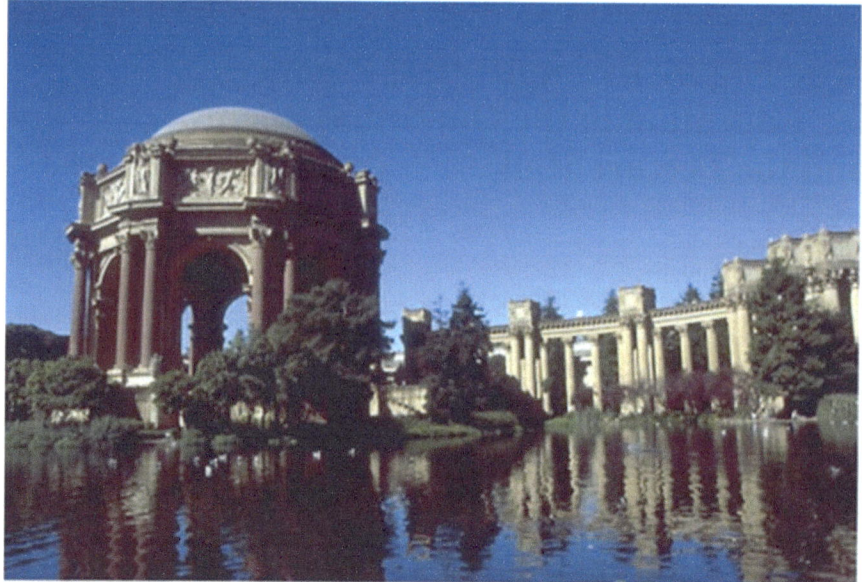

Fig. 2.1 The Exploratorium, housed in the Palace of Fine Arts in San Francisco. This building was constructed in 1915 for the Panama-Pacific World Exhibition and Fair

I learned communication, inquiry-based learning, and leadership skills without ever knowing that this is what I was being taught. We were always teaching, even when we were not aware of it, as we all watched and learned from each other, other students, and visitors alike. In the morning, we would meet before the doors opened to the public and often one of the full-time staff would go through one of the exhibits in detail with us so that we felt comfortable enough to explain it. I could not believe I was actually getting paid, albeit minimum wage, to learn and teach for 40 hours each week.

It is this philosophy, one of actively engaging the learner on his/her own terms and with real examples, that he/she can relate to that generates a lasting and functional knowledge. When education occurs in this way, with information presented in context, the learner is more able to grasp concepts that may seem foreign or strange if only discussed in theory. In this manner, the subject is not simply imparted as facts meant to be memorized and retrieved at the appropriate moment, but rather as facts placed in context. A rational approach to learning such as this provides the tools necessary to formulate and then answer questions that have not yet been asked. In the practice of clinical anesthesia, information is crucial. Decisions which quite literally have life or death consequences must be made quickly and with minimal hesitation. For knowledge to be useful under these circumstances, it must be transferred from the teacher to the learner in a purposeful context, so that it can be recalled under the appropriate circumstances and utilized by the learner.

Background

Graduate-level medical education differs from that which many students have experienced in the classroom [1]. Adult learners are self-directed and often work together in a mutual peer relationship with the teacher [2]. In the case of the anesthesia resident, this is often a very close relationship where one-on-one supervision and practical education is common, similar to that which occurs within the apprenticeship model. While children and young adult students require a set of directions that originate from the teacher, adult learners are more likely to initiate their own investigations, choosing some but not necessarily all of the educational opportunities available. In the field of anesthesiology, clinical teaching involves expanding the knowledge base (medicine, anatomy, pharmacology, physiology, etc.), practical training to develop psychomotor skills and abilities, and the imparting of many nonclinical aspects of anesthesia such as effective communication, leadership, management, and ethics [3]. A supervising anesthesiologist teaches a large portion of these required skills to resident physicians learning in the operating room (OR).

Everyone learns differently, and by the time the student has reached the level of graduate medical education, it is clear to him/her what works and what does not. These differences between learners tend to increase with age, and the graduate-level educator must take into account these differences when developing a personal style of teaching.

In the Operating Room

Despite the potential for a more personal interaction between attending anesthesiologist and resident, medical student, or student nurse anesthetist, the time factor for learning is especially crucial. Often the demands of the operating room schedule can seem to trump the need to illustrate a crucial point, elaborate on an event, or discuss an unexpected change in plans, but as will be discussed, this does not always have to be the case. To become an effective clinical teacher in the operating room environment takes a considerable amount of effort. These skills do not come naturally for everyone, but if a teenager with no formal background in physics and more than just a little stage fright can learn to explain physical phenomena to strangers, then I believe anyone can learn how to effectively educate the next generation of anesthesia care providers. There are specific actions that a teacher can take to more effectively transfer knowledge through modeling, demonstration, and example. Some of these actions are more obvious than others, but each is essential.

Making Time for Teaching

This requirement may seem intuitive, but given the ever-increasing demands placed on clinicians, even in the academic setting, it can seem less practical to devote time to nonclinical activity. It is often even difficult to arrange for attending physicians to be relieved from the clinical schedule to meet the basic educational requirements of a residency program. Some have even gone as far as to suggest that teaching in the OR may actually get in the way of maintaining an efficient operating room schedule [4, 5]. If the attending anesthesiologist takes the time to focus on teaching a resident or CRNA, makes a point of not moving forward until the learner has made a management decision, or allows them to attempt to manage the case in real time, the perception by the surgical and nursing staff can be that things are not moving along as quickly as they should, though one recent study suggests otherwise [6]. In this study only a moderate increase, a matter of minutes, was seen in the time to surgical incision when teaching of anesthesia residents was involved. In fact, the total contribution of resident education to total surgical time was less than 3 % of the total case time. As demands for increased efficiency continue to chip away at the limited time available for education, it should be remembered that every interaction must be seen as an opportunity to teach.

Often the demands of a busy clinical schedule do not provide the opportunity for lengthy discussions of clinical management strategies so it is helpful to have a number of short, prepared lessons to be used at opportune moments for a variety of purposes. These lessons can be used to focus a discussion on a particular topic, skill, or ability relevant to the current case. They may be used as an opportunity for the resident to break from the responsibility of actively managing the anesthetic, especially during a long period of clinical activity. If they are brief lessons which quickly make an effective point, they may be remembered more effectively by the resident than a lengthier lecture [7]. Examples of such lessons include management strategies for clinical scenarios which can be broadly applied such as emergency drugs for hypertensive crisis, developing a rapid differential diagnosis of intraoperative hypoxia, or even strategies for preventing postoperative nausea and vomiting.

When medical students were queried about behaviors considered exemplary and appropriate for positive attending physician role models, a simple willingness to take time for education is seen as an extremely positive attribute [8]. In July when the residents are in their first weeks of training in clinical anesthesia, finding time for education is relatively easy. Attending physicians are typically paired up with a single newly minted CA-1 and the entire day is devoted to education and training. It is in the months that follow when the residents find themselves "double-covered" and the attending's day involves covering multiple locations with simultaneous cases and coordinating lunch relief, coffee, and bathroom breaks that making time for teaching in the OR becomes an effort. It is during these busy hours when pausing for a few minutes to discuss a clinical point or putting aside a block of time for a well-thought-out mini-lecture or discussion in the afternoon can make a difference.

Creating an Appropriate Learning Environment

In addition to making plans to set aside time devoted to teaching during the day, residents need to know what is expected of them. We expect that residents will come to work prepared to perform clinically and that they will arrive prepared to actively participate in discussions related to these clinical activities. Unfortunately, we often do not take the time to make this clear or to provide the context for these discussions, and the end result is frustration in both parties.

Creating an appropriate learning environment starts with a clear statement of expectations. The call typically made by the resident to the attending they will be working with the evening before to discuss the following day's cases provides the ideal opportunity for an initial orientation. If the cases are complicated, then a plan to discuss specific related issues can be made at that time, giving the resident ample time to prepare. For example, if the schedule includes a particularly involved case or one that will be performed on a patient with significant comorbidities, the topic and context is clear. "We're performing a cholecystectomy tomorrow and even though this is a routine case the patient is on hemodialysis so why don't we discuss hyperkalemia tomorrow?" If the cases are routine, an offer to discuss a topic that the resident has been having trouble with or one he/she has questions about can underline the expectations that a discussion will occur at some point and that some preparation on the part of the resident is appropriate. Even if no formal plans have been made, every case presents an opportunity to discuss a particular topic.

During the days' cases the appropriate time for teaching will become clear. When the opportunity for discussion presents itself, it is helpful to physically position oneself in the room to have a full view of the patient and the monitors. The attending can both teach *and* supervise the case in progress at the same time. This is especially important for the resident learner who will need a "break" from the clinical management of the patient in order to focus attention on the teacher and the information presented. It is appropriate to pause as necessary to address patient care issues should they arise, but the resident or medical student should be focused on the discussion and not distracted by the need to adjust an infusion flow rate or re-dose a medication. If it is difficult for the learner to focus on the attending within the context of providing clinical care, specific data should be incorporated into the discussion. For example, if the lesson is a theoretical discussion of the different ways in which patients lose heat to the environment during anesthesia and the resident insists on adjusting the settings on the anesthesia delivery unit during the talk, then it should be emphasized how the flow rate and other settings can have a direct impact on patient temperature.

At the end of the day, it is essential that a "final evaluation" in the form of feedback be provided, along with recognition for the work that the resident has done throughout the day. An effective strategy is to end the day with a question. Asking the resident an open-ended question such as "how do you think you did today?" is often helpful. This will not only give the teacher a better idea of how well the lessons were received but also open the door to provide feedback and set the tone for future opportunities for learning.

Using Real-Life Examples

Medical schools are moving away from recruiting students with the classic undergraduate science background in favor of students with undergraduate backgrounds in the humanities. More and more medical students are now entering medical school without having had to take the Medical College Admission Test (MCAT) or the classic premed science courses. It can no longer be assumed that every resident will have a firm background in physics, chemistry, or even biology. The difference between theoretical and applied physics may be irrelevant to the anesthesia resident whose undergraduate studies did not include these topics, but by using examples that can be related to everyday experiences, one can effectively illustrate a point and influence students to adopt appropriate clinical management choices.

Since the issue of heat loss came up in the last section, an example here is appropriate. Heat loss is a basic topic that is covered in most high school physics courses, so the assumption that this is not new information is likely correct. What *is* new is the context in which this information is being presented. For the first time, the student is being asked to recall basic understanding of the physics of heat transfer and apply it to a clinical situation, using that information to intervene in a manner which appropriately prevents the transfer of heat from the patient to the environment. While most residents will not be able to discuss the concepts of conduction, convection, evaporation, and radiation in scientific terms (though some may) once they are reminded of information they already know, they will become actively engaged in the learning process.

One might begin the discussion by talking about the weather. Is it cold outside today? Why does one feel cold when one walks outside? Through what mechanisms is heat transferred away from the body in this context? Where does it go? Is it windy today? Why does that make it feel colder than it actually is? And then one might ask "How can we take advantage of these phenomena to prevent heat transfer or actively warm patients?" It is likely that every resident has taken a shower before, possibly even on the day of this discussion. One might ask then what happens when a person steps out of the shower into the bathroom? Why does one feel cold? The resident might not remember the actual value for the heat of vaporization for water[1], but anyone who has experienced this and started shivering knows intuitively that it is a significant value. Now one might continue by asking "What happens when the ability to increase temperature by shivering is removed in the patient who is now paralyzed?" "How does the vasodilation that occurs when the patient is under the influence of anesthetic vapors effect temperature?" or "If a significant body surface area is washed with a cold liquid antiseptic how does that contribute to heat loss?"

Making It Interesting and Including Emotional Content

Almost everyone remembers where they were on September 11, 2001, when we first learned about the terrorists' attacks on the World Trade Center in New York and on the Pentagon in Washington, DC. Chances are that the moments are recalled in

---

[1] The heat of vaporization or heat of evaporation (enthalpy of vaporization) is the energy required to transform a given quantity of a substance from a liquid into a gas at a given pressure (often atmospheric pressure). Heat is lost and you feel cold when energy is used to facilitate the evaporation of water off your skin.

vivid detail including the room where one was when the first news reports appeared on television. One might very well remember who was and who was not present in that room and maybe even remember the clothes that he/she was wearing. But if one tries to recall those same details for September 11, 2000, there are likely no or at least very scant memories. Emotional arousal has been shown to enhance one or more memory stages, including the creation of new memories (encoding), the persistence of memories (consolidation), and the final access to stored information (retrieval) [9]. As compared to typical memories which rely upon hippocampal pathways, events associated with high emotional content and anxiety are fixed in human memory via pathways that involve the amygdala [10, 11].

This theory was applied clinically in an elegant study designed to improve the retention of Advanced Cardiac Life Support (ACLS) skills taught to medical students by adding emotional content to the ACLS course [12]. Medical students who had not previously taken an ACLS course were recruited to participate in this study. All of the students attended the didactic portion of the course and then were randomly assigned to one of two groups, experimental or control, for the practical portion of the course. Students in the experimental (emotional content) group experienced the Megacode portion of the course in full-environment simulation (FES) with realistic simulation equipment and actors playing ancillary personnel. A significant amount of realism designed to increase the stress level of participants (validated by statistically increased heart rate and self-reported anxiety inventory) was part of the experimental group's experience. Students in the control group experienced the Megacode portion of the course without the increased realism or stress. Students in the experimental group demonstrated a statistically significant improvement during Megacode performance 6 months after the course. The authors suggested that this improved recall was related to the manner in which the information was initially encoded.

Though this experiment was conducted in a state of the art simulator center and required considerable resources, it is not necessary to go to such expense to take advantage of this theory. Simply adding emotional content to a story can improve the ability of the listener to recall specific details that they would otherwise not remember [13]. Educational experiences in the operating room combine visual and auditory learning based in real time with emotional sensations allowing trainees to develop a "clinical memory" [14]. In this way, the presentation of otherwise dry information in a context which provides relevance and engages the learner on many levels can not only improve the overall experience for the teacher but also improve student recall [2].

When learning occurs in the high-stakes context of the operating room environment, the emotional context of this setting alone can enhance learning. Often the experience of making a mistake that results in a near-miss or in actual patient harm is stressful enough to ensure that the learner never duplicates the error. The anesthesia care provider who cannot recall administering the wrong medication to a patient either is not paying attention, has not practiced clinically for very long, or is being disingenuous. While such mistakes should never happen in clinical practice, there is no denying the impact they have on a clinician's practice. We remember from our failures not our successes, and it is these events that (sometimes) end with an untoward outcome that create "seasoned" veteran clinicians.

Encouraging the Learner to Teach Juniors

The most effective demonstration of concept mastery is the ability to explain the topic to someone else. It is in this context that the old rubric of "see one, do one, teach one" remains appropriate. The student who understands well enough to explain differently the concept that he or she has just learned demonstrates a deeper understanding, more than a simple ability to repeat what has simply been heard. Knowledge is assimilated, in part, when the learner must reform the information in his or her own mind so that it may be presented to the student. Senior residents should be encouraged to actively participate in the education of junior residents and medical students rotating through the department. Developing this depth of understanding is critical to the creation of both the next generation of educators and the next generation of clinicians.

Though the majority of anesthesia residents will not end up in an academic practice setting, every single one of them will be tasked with educating their surgical and nursing colleagues as well as their future patients. The ability to clearly explain the pertinent issues at hand has more than once avoided medical catastrophe and alleviated anxiety during crises when adverse outcomes have occurred.

Encouraging Students to Question What They Are Taught

Research suggests that it is often difficult to ask questions, especially when such questions might be seen as a challenge to the knowledge or expertise of "superiors" [15, 16]. Early training in anesthesiology can be somewhat overwhelming as residents are asked to perform in an environment unlike one they have ever experienced before. There is a steep learning curve involved as residents struggle to master the technical skills required to safely administer an anesthetic while at the same time attending to the tasks associated with record keeping and maintaining regulation compliance. It can be very easy for the resident in this position to just let the attending plan the anesthetic without question in order to make the day go smoother, but this approach does not develop the critical thinking skills that the resident will absolutely need to have mastered by the time of graduation in a few short years.

There are many different ways to provide safe and effective anesthesia for any given procedure and patient, and this point should be emphasized to junior residents. They should be encouraged to constantly ask "why?" when they are told by an attending to do something a certain way. The first time I work with a resident, after we have determined how we are going to administer anesthesia for the first case of the day, I make the following comment: "This is the way I do it, it is by no means the only way and though I think it is the best way to provide anesthesia to this patient for this case you are allowed to disagree. Your job over the next 3 years is to take whatever methods and tricks that you are taught and incorporate them to produce your own style. You may find that you like some of what I do and combine that with some things that others do, but to effectively do this you need to constantly question why the anesthesiologists you work with choose to do things the way they do".

When I am working alone, I provide anesthesia the way I prefer to, but when I am supervising a resident, the choice is less clear and should be arrived at by discussion. Provided the anesthetic is safe, effective, and does not harm the patient and the resident can communicate a rationale for the choices that have been made, I will allow him or her to dictate the type of anesthesia to be administered. Providing increased opportunities for resident success (and failure), sharing responsibility for developing the anesthetic plan, and encouraging residents to overcome communication barriers within the medical hierarchy are essential parts of education in the operating room [17].

Classroom Teaching

Medicine is in many ways an applied science and anesthesiology is even more so. As we have seen, this makes it particularly well suited for learning at the bedside while in the operating room. Still, there is some place for introduction of basic information or discussion of classic problems, and the opportunity for a discussion between larger groups without the distractions of patient care does present some advantages. Despite the considerable evidence that the use of simulation techniques to educate medical professionals is effective [18] and a move away from the traditional classroom setting for medical education [19], studies have shown that even for developing skills related to clinical situations, the classroom setting is still an appropriate and worthwhile venue [20]. Most residency programs present didactic material in the classroom setting to ensure consistency in the content delivered to their residents, but just as some attending physicians are better at teaching at the bedside than their peers, some are better at presenting didactic material in the classroom.

We have all been through the "grand rounds" lecture or classroom presentation that it seemed would never end. Despite being delivered by the "world's expert" on the particular topic, the presentation seemed to be more effective as an anesthetic induction agent than a vehicle for the delivery of new information. Looking around it was clear that the majority of people in the audience had entered a state similar to general anesthesia well before the halfway point. What is it that makes some lectures more effective than others? Is it the content of the lecture or the presentation? In many ways it is both. There are some presenters that can make even the driest material seem interesting and others that are quite skilled at making the most interesting topics seem dry. A careful examination of the practices that are most effective follows.

Know Your Audience

The most effective presenters have the ability to tailor their presentation to the level of comprehension their audience is likely capable of while at the same time meeting their individual needs. The expert in anesthetic pharmacology who is presenting new and exciting information on drug discovery to an entire anesthesia department should remember that the audience will consist of residents at different levels of training, SRNA and CRNAs, and attending physicians, many of whom are not themselves involved in drug discovery and are not at all interested in the intricacies of the scientific process relating to this issue. The effective classroom presenter is able to give the same lecture to a range of different audiences without losing students along the way. Resident-level classroom sessions are much different than mixed audience grand rounds presentations or even industry-sponsored meeting presentations, and the effective lecturer must know his or her audience before beginning to speak.

Length Matters

Presenting material effectively depends on keeping the attention of your audience. For most topics, the less time you spend on them, the more likely your audience will be able to follow what you are saying and keep their attention focused on your presentation. Most classroom sessions are to be conducted within a specific preset period of time, so while you likely don't have the option of running over time, it is possible to truncate your presentation, leaving time for questions, discussion, or clarification at the end of the talk. When there is a significant amount of material that needs to be presented, consider either editing the lecture to focus only on the high points or breaking the material up into two (or more) lectures to be delivered on different days.

Using Slides

A picture is worth far more than a thousand words; it is also worth the time it takes to describe the image; and in the classroom setting with attentions waning, time is precious. The judicious use of slides to present material can save both the time required to describe complicated topics or material and the time required for clarification thereof. The effective classroom teacher uses slides to keep the audience of students focused on the topic. The slides should contain information that the presenter is actively presenting. The presenter should not simply read the information on the slides. The slides should contain relevant and related information that the students can refer to while listening to the presentation. Slides which complement the presentation rather than duplicate the information being taught are much more effective than a simple visual transcript of the lecture. If you have problems remembering what you had planned to say, slides should not be used as a transcript but instead notes or other cues should be considered.

Audience Participation

Some topics lend themselves to audience participation better than others, and some audiences participate more effectively than others. It is important to strike a balance between asking too many questions and not enough requests for participation. Simply presenting the material without requesting verbal conformation that anyone is listening is as bad as spending more time asking questions (especially if nobody is answering) than covering the required material. The most effective presenters can gauge the response of the audience and adjust requests for participation as needed. Questions peppered throughout the presentation at appropriate intervals can be a very effective way of maintaining audience attention. If the students know that at any moment they might be asked a question based on the material that was just presented or, even better, be asked to use this new information to answer a related question, then it is more likely that they will be actively following the lecture as it evolves. The use of computer-generated responses is also an effective, if rather expensive, means to education. In this scenario, participants are not singled out but rather can express their opinion with the rest of the audience and then realize the expression of the majority.

Conclusion

We as attending physicians in academic practice are tasked with keeping "one step ahead" of our residents, and these students seem to be getting smarter and smarter every year. As new medical devices and therapies are brought into clinical practice, we may even find ourselves learning new techniques alongside or in some cases from our juniors. But more important than demonstrating clinical excellence or facility with the latest device is the role modeling that takes place at the patients' "bedside" in the operating room. It is this demonstration of how to effectively manage any situation, regardless of the intensity of the crisis or the severity of the risk involved, that most will remember and (hopefully) strive to emulate. In this context, academics and attendings are always "teaching." Every comment uttered or behavior exhibited has the potential to affect the development of the next generation of attending physicians.

References

1. Schwind CJ, Boehler ML, Rogers DA, et al. Variables influencing medical student learning in the operating room. Am J Surg. 2004;187:198–200.
2. Lyon PMA. Making the most of learning in the operating theatre: student strategies and curricular initiatives. Med Educ. 2003;37:680–8.
3. Jones RW, Morris RW. Facilitating learning in the operating theatre and intensive care unit. Anaesth Intensive Care. 2006;34(6):758–64.

4. Hanss R, Roemer T, Hedderich J, Roesler L, Steinfath M, Bein B, et al. Influence of anaesthesia resident training on the duration of three common surgical operations. Anaesthesia. 2009;64(6):632–7.
5. Schuster M, Kotjan T, Fiege M, Goetz AE. Influence of resident training on anaesthesia induction times. Br J Anaesth. 2008;101(5):640–7.
6. Davis EA, Escobar A, Ehrenwerth J, Watrous GA, Fisch GS, Kain ZN, et al. Resident teaching versus the operating room schedule: an independent observer-based study of 1558 cases. Anesth Analg. 2006;103(4):932–7.
7. Mason RA. Education and training in airway management. Br J Anaesth. 1998;81:305–7.
8. Curry SE, Courtland CI, Graham MJ. Role-modelling in the operating room: medical student observations of exemplary behaviour. Med Educ. 2011;45:946–57.
9. Dolcos F, LaBar KS, Cabeza R. Remembering one year later: role of the amygdala and the medial temporal lobe memory system in retrieving emotional memories. Proc Natl Acad Sci U S A. 2005;102(7):2626–31.
10. Cahill L, Haier RJ, Fallon J, Alkire MT, Tang C, Keator D, et al. Amygdala activity at encoding correlated with long-term, free recall of emotional information. Proc Natl Acad Sci U S A. 1996;93:8016–21.
11. Sandi C, Pinelo-Nava MT. Stress and memory: behavioral effects and neurobiological mechanisms. Neural Plast. 2007;2007:78970.
12. DeMaria Jr S, Bryson EO, Mooney TJ, Silverstein JH, Reich DL, Bodian C, et al. Adding emotional stressors to training in simulated cardiopulmonary arrest enhances participant performance. Med Educ. 2010;44(10):1006–15.
13. Cahill L. The neurobiology of emotionally influenced memory. Implications for understanding traumatic memory. Ann N Y Acad Sci. 1997;821:238–46.
14. Cox K. Teaching and learning clinical perception. Med Educ. 1996;30:90–6.
15. Crosskerry P. The feedback sanction. Acad Emerg Med. 2000;7:1232–8.
16. Milgram S. Behavioral study of obedience. J Abnorm Psychol. 1963;67:371–8.
17. Pian-Smith MC, Simon R, Minehart RD, Podraza M, Rudolph J, Walzer T, et al. Teaching residents the two-challenge rule: a simulation-based approach to improve education and patient safety. Simul Healthc. 2009;4(2):84–91.
18. Okuda H, Bryson EO, DeMaria Jr S, Jacobson L, Quinones J, Shen B, et al. The utility of simulation in medical education: what is the evidence? Mt Sinai J Med. 2009;76(4):330–43.
19. Sherbino J, Chan T, Schiff K. The reverse classroom: lectures on your own and homework with faculty. CJEM. 2013;15(3):178–80.
20. Clay-Williams R, McIntosh CA, Kerridge R, Braithwaite J. Classroom and simulation team training: a randomized controlled trial. Int J Qual Health Care. 2013;25(3):314–21.

Chapter 3
Learning from Incident Reporting and Closed Claims Analyses

Julia Metzner, Karen L. Posner, and Karen B. Domino

Abbreviations

AIRS	Anesthesia incident reporting system
ASA	American Society of Anesthesiologists
CIR	Critical incident reporting
L/min	Liters per minute
MAC	Monitored anesthesia care
NACOR	National Anesthesia Clinical Outcomes Registry
O_2	Oxygen
OR	Operating room
OSA	Obstructive sleep apnea
PACU	Postanesthesia care unit
RCA	Root cause analysis
TOF	Train of four

Developing a superior understanding of medical errors that represent a threat to patient safety and implementing measures to reduce patient risk are fundamental goals of modern health care systems. Anesthesiologists were focused on patient safety well before the landmark Institute of Medicine Report, "To Err is Human," was released in November 1999 [1]. This landmark report cited the specialty of anesthesia as among the most effective specialties to reduce the incidence of untoward events: a decrease in mortality rates from two deaths/10,000 anesthetics administered, to one death/200,000–300,000 anesthetics administered [2]. Although these achievements are impressive, anesthetic mishaps still do happen, commonly related

---

J. Metzner, M.D. • K.L. Posner, Ph.D. • K.B. Domino, M.D., M.P.H. (✉)
Department of Anesthesiology and Pain Medicine, University of Washington,
1959 NE Pacific Street, BB 1431, Seattle, WA 98195-6540, USA
e-mail: metznj@uw.edu; posner@uw.edu; kdomino@uw.edu

to lack of knowledge, teamwork, or communication, systems failure, and human errors. Capturing infrequently occurring adverse events is extremely difficult, and this is why patient safety reporting systems both at the local and national level are essential. This chapter will highlight the importance of critical incident reporting and the role of the American Society of Anesthesiologists (ASA) Closed Claims Project as indispensable tools to identify, analyze, and rectify problems in the delivery of care.

Critical Incidents Reporting

Critical incidents reporting (CIR) was originally developed in the aircraft industry as a method to improve safety and performance during military applications. The model was very quickly integrated into anesthesiology quality improvement programs [3]. By definition, a critical incident is any event or condition that led or could have led to patient harm (if not intercepted, e.g., a "near-miss"). Within US hospitals, CIR is usually initiated by care providers (doctors, nurses), risk management, or other administrative bodies. Reporting systems may also be designed to receive information from patients, families, or consumer advocates.

It is critical that reporting be confidential, non-punitive, and protected from legal discovery. The desire to improve patient safety should surpass the fear of the penalty of reporting. CIR is of highest value when it promotes learning from mistakes and leads to a constructive response that will mitigate these hazards to patient safety [4]. Within a health care institution, reporting of a serious event or serious "near-miss" should trigger an in-depth investigation or root cause analysis (RCA) to identify underlying system failures that can lead to system redesign in order to prevent recurrence.

Root Cause Analysis

RCA is a systematic approach to pin down step-by-step the causal factors and essentially dig into the roots of a critical incident (Fig. 3.1). As a general rule, RCA includes investigation of both active errors (errors occurring at the point of interface between provider actions and complex systems) and latent errors (the breakdowns or system flaws within health care systems that contribute to undesirable events) contributing to the critical incident. The goal of RCA is to develop an action plan to implement system changes that will potentially prevent recurrence of similar incidents in the future.

The RCA first determines *what* happened by recreating the sequence of events in chronological order and, without being judgmental, *how* the critical event occurred by comparing the sequence of events to the ideal intended process flow. This analytic step will reveal system flaws and/or human errors in the sequence of events leading to the critical incident. This step may reveal omissions made by the staff involved in the care, as well as insight into the chain of events which set up the conditions for the incident to occur. The next step in the analysis is assessing *why* errors occurred.

3 Learning from Incident Reporting and Closed Claims Analyses

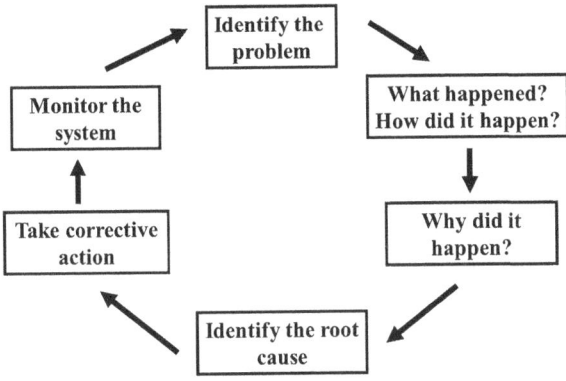

Fig. 3.1 Steps of root cause analysis

Table 3.1 Contributory factors leading to an incident

Contributory factors	Examples
Human performance	Lack of knowledge or skills at individual level; inadequate training; performance pressure; failure to monitor, observe, or act.
Organization	Missing protocols or defective guidelines, lack of resources and support. Selection, training, and credentialing; performance assessments; scheduling, staff assignment aligned with training/experience.
Team communication	Preoperative checklist procedures; incomplete handoff.
Environment/equipment	Equipment not maintained per schedule; missing items from anesthesia cart; no standardized location for emergency equipment.

This process analyzes the comparison between the ideal and actual process flow leading to the incident for factors contributing to the mismatch between ideal and actual process flow (Table 3.1). Contributory factors such as lack of knowledge or training at the individual level, missing protocols at the task level, poor communication at the team level, or inadequate staffing at the organizational level should be explored. Specific contributory factors should be distinguished from, or studied in context with, general contributory factors such as poor safety culture within the system, communication failure, poor training, overstretched scheduling, or defective guidelines. The final step in RCA is development of an *action plan* to correct system flaws and prevent future errors identified in the RCA. The plan is then *implemented and monitored* through quality improvement procedures.

A Meaningful RCA Should Generally Follow These Basic Steps

Step 1: Assemble a multidisciplinary RCA team
- Team members include physicians, nurses, technicians, administrators, and any other personnel directly involved in the chain of events.
- Nominate a team leader with expertise in RCA investigation.

Step 2: Dig into the roots to understand WHAT HAPPENED and HOW IT HAPPENED

- Generate an accurate chronology of events.
- Gather the facts using documents, medical records, and staff interviews.
- Review relevant policy and procedure standards.
- Generate an ideal process flow map.
- Compare actual sequence of events with internal policy or evidence-based practice according to literature or guidelines.

Step 3: Identify root causes: WHY DID IT HAPPEN?

- Identify discrepancies between ideal process flow and actual sequence of events.
- Determine the contributory factors that lead to the incident (Table 3.1).
- Identify system factors that may contribute to individual performance deficits.
- Identify and summarize both active and latent errors.

Step 4: Develop an action plan: WHAT CAN BE DONE TO PREVENT IT FROM HAPPENING AGAIN?

- Based on RCA analysis, make feasible recommendations to fix the system: change policies, refresh practice guidelines, redesign the process.
- Nominate the individual(s) who will be accountable for the implementation and monitoring of recommendations (system owner).
- Determine a time-frame for implementation.
- Pilot test system changes.
- Evaluate the results of the action plan and system redesign.

Step 5: Monitor the effectiveness of the action plan

- Decrease in the risk of occurrence.
- Follow-up reviews for plan contingency.

Incident Reporting Can Be a Source of Transmitted Learning

Critical incidents and "near miss" reporting can be a powerful tool for developing and maintaining an awareness of risks in anesthesiology practice. Anesthesia registries, such as the National Anesthesia Clinical Outcomes Registry (NACOR), and the Anesthesia Incident Reporting System (AIRS) represent national web-based CIR systems to gather data on adverse events and outcomes [5]. The AIRS (aqihq.org) publishes analysis of critical incident cases monthly in the ASA Newsletter.

The ASA Closed Claims Project investigates anesthesia adverse events and outcomes using closed malpractice insurance claim files [6]. The Closed Claims Project database is a standardized collection of >10,000 cases retrieved from the closed claim files of medical liability insurers throughout the USA. Analysis of malpractice claims offers a unique opportunity to understand how critical incidents contribute to the genesis of adverse outcomes [7].

3 Learning from Incident Reporting and Closed Claims Analyses

We picked two cases from the Closed Claims Project database to illustrate analysis of adverse events using a RCA: an operating room fire and a failed extubation with difficult reintubation. Some details have been changed to protect confidentiality. RCA examples are abbreviated to illustrate selected parts of the RCA process for each case example.

Critical Incident #1: Fire in the Operating Room (OR)

A 53-year-old, ASA 3 obese female (91 kg) with history of chronic lymphocytic leukemia, asthma, and depression underwent a cervical lymph node biopsy under monitored anesthesia care (MAC) with sedation. A simple facemask was applied to the patient's face with oxygen (O_2), flowing at 7 L/min. The surgical site was prepped with an alcohol/iodine solution and then sterile disposable paper drapes were placed over the field, which also covered the patient's face and her oxygen mask. Following incision, the surgeon used an electrocautery to provide hemostasis at the surgical edges. A sudden flash fire started on the neck area with rapid propagation to the paper drapes and the oxygen mask. The anesthesiologist promptly turned the oxygen flowmeter off, and then swiftly removed the face mask; simultaneously the drapes were pulled off and the ignition area soaked with 0.9% saline. Although the fire was quickly extinguished, the patient suffered superficial burns to her neck and perinasal area, and singed eyebrows. The burn injuries were locally treated and the surgery was completed. The patient was admitted overnight and then discharged home the next day after disclosure of the events.

RCA Framework

What Happened?

Table 3.2 illustrates a condensed sequence of events, including deficiencies in the process flow, and examples of action plans that could be adopted to correct these deficiencies.

Chronological Sequence of Events

1. Minimally invasive surgery on the neck under MAC with sedation
2. Surgical field cleaned with alcohol-based solution
3. High flow of O_2 administered under paper drapes
4. Surgical electrocautery used which started a fire
5. Despite prompt team interaction to stop the fire, patient suffered burn injuries

Why Did It Happen? What Steps Were Contributory to the Event?

The RCA committee performed an in-depth analysis of the critical incident and outlined the following contributory factors that lead to this adverse outcome.

Table 3.2 Fire in the OR—root cause analysis

Chronological sequence of events (what happened? How did it happen?)	Identification of root causes/ contributory factors (why did it happen?)	Action plan: prevention of recurrence
Surgery on the neck under MAC with O_2 by facemask	High fire-risk surgery	Compile and distribute a list of high fire-risk procedures
		Educate staff to recognize a fire triad
Area prepped with alcohol-based solution	The OR team failed to recognize the presence of a fire triad (fuel, oxidizer, ignition source)	Include fire hazard in the Universal Protocol and time-out
Face mask with high oxygen flow under paper drapes	Lack of communication	Institute team communication training
Electrocautery activated with initiation of a fire	Lack of preventive measures at hospital and individual level	Develop clear fire precaution protocols
	Lack of proper education and training	Periodically rehearse knowledge and awareness
Burning materials promptly removed from patient, and involved area doused with saline	Management of on-patient fire was appropriate	While fire management was appropriate once it occurred, given the institutional lack of fire safety awareness, fire management should be included in education and protocols

OR operating room, *MAC* monitored anesthesia care, O_2 oxygen

Factors Relevant to the Outcome

I. Active errors related to human factors:
  A. OR team failed to identify a high-risk fire situation (Fig. 3.2)
     In order for an intraoperative fire to occur, all the key elements of the fire triad must be present including ignition source (electrocautery, laser, etc.), fuel (paper or plastic drapes, gauze, airway devices, patient's hair, etc.), and an oxidizer (oxygen, nitrous-oxide).
  B. No strategies applied to prevent the risk of fire
     1. Lack of communication between care providers: the surgeon should have announced that he planned to use electrocoagulation; the anesthesiologist should have alerted the surgeon about the existence of a high O_2 source in the field.
     2. Inefficient fire safety plan structure: surgical drapes should be configured in a manner to minimize the accumulation of oxygen under the drapes; flammable prepping solutions should be left to dry 3 min before draping; moist or wet gauzes/sponges should be used for high fire-risk surgeries; flow of O_2 should be reduced to minimum or ceased for a few minutes before electrocautery.

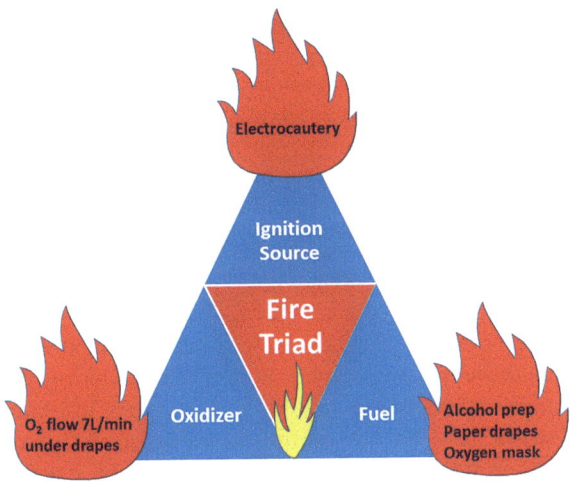

Fig. 3.2 Fire triad involves ignition source, oxidizer, and fuel. Specific elements of the triad from the case example are shown. *O₂* oxygen, *L/min* liters per minute

II. Latent errors related to system failures

   A. Awareness and prevention strategies for surgical fires were unavailable at the hospital level.
   B. Insufficient level of training and education of OR staff related to risk of intraoperative fire and safety issues.

What Can Be Done to Prevent It from Happening Again? What Preventive Measures Should Be Taken?

1. Provide a list of high fire-risk procedures
2. Preoperative checklist with steps to prevent fire
3. Foster open communication between OR team members for high fire-risk procedures

Action Plan

1. Develop hospital-specific fire prevention algorithm with inclusion of fire risk in the preoperative checklist
2. Develop hospital-specific fire management plan
3. Regular practice of fire drills

RCA Summary of Events

The case involved an oncologic patient for lymph node biopsy under MAC anesthesia. Upon activation of electrocautery on alcohol-based surgical prep in an oxygen-enriched environment, the paper drapes and facemask caught on fire. The fire was promptly extinguished; however, the patient suffered burn injuries. The RCA committee agreed that lack of awareness for potential fire, poor communication, and lack of standard safety precautions played a major role in this serious adverse outcome.

Case Discussion

Surgical fires in the OR are rare events, but if a fire occurs it can result in dire consequences for the patients, care providers, and hospital. This closed claims case could easily occur in any OR when the well-known components of a fire triad are present and fire prevention plans are lacking. The case mirrors the findings of a recent closed claims malpractice review [8] that analyzed 103 fire claims which occurred between 1985 and 2009. Most fire claims occurred in patients receiving MAC for surgeries on the head, neck, and upper torso. Most (90 %) fires were ignited by electrocautery. Supplemental 100 % O_2, with an open delivery system (rather than endotracheal tube or laryngeal mask airway), was present in nearly all of the cases. In contrast, alcohol-containing preps were used in only a minority of these cases. While most fires resulted in superficial burns, some did result in severe injury or death, and the majority of these malpractice claims resulted in compensation to the patient.

The risk of fires in the operating room has been recognized for over 60 years [9, 10]. There are extensive resources available to provide guidance in OR fire safety, including a practice advisory by the ASA [11]. The ASA practice advisory provides guidance on fire preparedness and prevention, as well as fire management should an operating room fire occur. Central to fire prevention in a high fire-risk procedure is communication within the surgery team and an agreed-upon fire prevention plan at the start of the procedure. A checklist for management of operating room fires is available [12]. Checklists have been shown to be effective for team management of relatively rare crises that occur in the OR [13].

Critical Incident #2: Failed Extubation with Difficult Reintubation

A 30-year-old obese (body mass index 38) male presented for a Le Fort I procedure with arch bar to treat his obstructive sleep apnea (OSA) symptoms. In anticipation of a difficult intubation, the anesthesia team elected to conduct asleep nasal fiberoptic intubation, which was easily performed. General anesthesia was administered for 6 h without problems. At the end of the case, the train of four (TOF) twitch response was assessed as inadequate for reversal of neuromuscular blockade, so the patient was taken to postanesthesia care unit (PACU) intubated. Ten minutes later, the patient had his eyes open and was sitting upright with good tidal volume, coughing violently from the endotracheal tube. Without performing airway suctioning or another TOF check, the anesthesiologist immediately removed the tube.

3 Learning from Incident Reporting and Closed Claims Analyses

About 30–40 s after extubation, the patient coughed up blood and his airway became obstructed. It was impossible to insert an oral airway due to swelling and copious bleeding. A nasal airway was placed, but bag-mask ventilation proved to be difficult. Surgical assistance and emergency difficult airway equipment were requested. During this period, the patient's oxygen saturation ranged between 66 and 80% and later became undetectable. Approximately 10–15 min after extubation, the surgeon arrived and performed a stat tracheostomy. The patient suffered hypoxic encephalopathy and died on the fourth postoperative day.

RCA Framework

What Happened?

Table 3.3 illustrates a condensed sequence of events, including deficiencies in the process flow, and example action plans that could be adopted to correct these deficiencies.

Chronological Sequence of Events

1. Patient did not meet extubation criteria in OR so transported to PACU intubated
2. Tracheal tube removal (extubation) without rechecking extubation criteria
3. Extubation failure in PACU in a patient with perioperatively compromised airway
4. Consequent loss of upper airway patency and "can't oxygenate/ventilate" airway emergency
5. Emergency surgical airway summoned
6. Airway reestablished by surgical intervention
7. Death resulting from hypoxic ischemic encephalopathy

Why Did It Happen? What Steps Were Contributory to the Event?

The RCA committee performed an in-depth analysis and outlined the following contributory factors that lead to this disastrous outcome.

Factors Relevant to the Outcome

I. Active errors related to human factors:
   A. Error of planning and executing: inadequate strategy for safe extubation and failure to recognize the potential of post-extubation difficult airway.
      Although the preoperative history of this patient (obesity, OSA) prompted the providers to consider potential difficulty in airway management, considerations for difficult extubation were omitted, and consequently no extubation plan was in place.

Table 3.3 Failed extubation root cause analysis

Chronological sequence of events (what happened? How did it happen?)	Identification of root causes/contributory factors (why did it happen?)	Action plan: prevention of recurrence
Anticipated difficult intubation	Intubation plan followed existing protocol for anticipated difficult airway	No action plan required
	Process deviation: Anesthesia team did not have a predetermined extubation plan	Difficult Airway Alert to follow patient from preop through PACU with difficult airway checklist to include intubation contingency plans, difficult airway cart in OR and PACU, extubation plan, availability of backup personnel including surgical airway
Patient did not meet extubation criteria in OR so transported to PACU intubated	*Process deviation*: None	Difficult airway alert as above
	Patient extubation status appropriately checked with TOF; acceptable to transport patient intubated to PACU	
	Contributory factors: Production pressure to move patient out of OR	Revise OR scheduling protocol and staffing to reduce production pressure
Patient extubated in the PACU	*Process deviation*: Anesthesia team did not reevaluate extubation criteria (TOF), did not suction airway prior to extubation	Extubation checklist for all patients who arrive intubated to PACU to be included in Difficult Airway Alert
Failed extubation in the PACU of a difficult airway with consecutive airway obstruction and inability to oxygenate/ventilate	*Process deviation*: Failure to implement safety measures for difficult extubation, i.e., use of an airway exchange catheter, surgeon at the bedside ready for surgical airway, difficult airway equipment available	Extubation checklist in Difficult Airway Alert to include these items
	Contributory factors: (Latent errors) Recovery staff not prepared for difficult airway management	In-service training for PACU staff including simulation training
	Difficult airway equipment not readily available	PACU difficult airway cart ready and regularly checked
	Process deviation: (Active errors) Failed to attempt different emergency airway management techniques	ASA Difficult Airway Algorithm
Emergency surgical airway requested with stat tracheotomy/cricothyrotomy performed by the surgeon	(Latent errors) Surgical support not immediately available	Staffing assignments to assure surgical staff availability for airway emergencies in OR or PACU
	Contributory factor: (Latent errors) Recovery staff not prepared for emergency surgical airway	Difficult airway drill in the simulator center

PACU postanesthesia care unit, *OR* operating room, *TOF* train of four, *ASA* American Society of Anesthesiologists

1. Deviations from standard at extubation:
    a. Did not monitor the adequacy of muscle strength (TOF)
    b. The airway was not suctioned and cleared from secretions
2. Insufficient preparation for a difficult extubation
    a. Backup airway equipment (difficult airway cart) was not readily available
    b. Surgeon not at bedside ready for an emergent surgical airway
    c. Agents to break laryngospasm (succinylcholine, propofol) not readily available
    d. Did not consider alternative interventions to secure the airway: e.g., tube exchange catheter, direct laryngoscopy, video-laryngoscopy (e.g., GlideScope®), or fast-track laryngeal mask airway
  B. Failure to follow established protocols:
    1. In the situation of cannot oxygenate and ventilate, the ASA Practice Guidelines for Management of the Difficult Airway [14] should be followed.
II. Latent errors related to system failures
  A. Recovery unit (PACU) poorly prepared for emergent management of difficult airway
  B. Limited PACU staff knowledge about the existence and location of emergency airway cart
  C. Surgeon not immediately available to provide emergency surgical airway
  D. PACU staff not trained to provide assistance for emergency surgical airway
III. Production pressure
  A. Anesthesia team: need to move patient to PACU to provide OR availability
  B. Anesthesia team: need to extubate patient for PACU handoff and be available to start the next case
  C. PACU staff: workload concerns for the management of an intubated patient

What Can Be Done to Prevent It from Happening Again? What Preventive Measures Should Be Taken?

1. Human performance: reinforce extubation rules and the ASA Difficult Airway Algorithm [14] for "cannot ventilate" situations
2. Communication breakdown: prepare the surgeon and facilitative staff for emergent airway management

3. Technological support: train providers to use alternative methods to secure the airway; make sure that staff has been adequately trained in the use of available equipment
4. Environmental aspects: assure that work area (PACU) supports handling a difficult airway (i.e., space, competency, safety, access)

Action Plan

1. Difficult airway drill in the simulation center
2. Checklists for extubation of the difficult airway
3. Reassessment of cognitive and technical performance
4. Periodical performance testing

RCA Summary of Events

An obese patient with obstructive sleep apnea (OSA) suffered failed extubation in the PACU. The preoperative history (obesity, OSA) and nature of the surgery should have suggested potential difficulty in airway management; the problem was most probably laryngospasm with blood clot and consecutive airway obstruction. The anesthesia providers should have anticipated this problem and prepared for the extubation of a difficult airway. Numerous systems issues represented latent errors that contributed to the adverse outcome for this patient.

Case Discussion

Complications associated with respiratory system management accounted for 17 % of surgical anesthesia claims in 1990–2007 [6]. Difficult intubation was the most common respiratory system event leading to anesthesia malpractice claims. Claims associated with difficult tracheal intubation have been increasing as a proportion of respiratory events leading to malpractice claims, accounting for 27 % of respiratory-related malpractice claims in 1990–2007 [6].

The ASA first introduced formal guidelines for management of the difficult airway in 1993 [15]. These have been updated periodically, with the most recent update in 2013 [14]. Data from the ASA Closed Claims Project was utilized to evaluate changes in difficult airway claims that might reflect changes in practice after initial guideline adoption [16]. While death or severe brain damage resulted in greater than half of difficult airway claims, there was a significant reduction in these outcomes associated with difficult intubation at induction of anesthesia after adoption of the difficult airway guidelines [16]. Unfortunately, there was no similar reduction in poor outcome following failed extubation. Similar to this case, difficult mask ventilation and development of an airway emergency were associated with poor outcome [16, 17]. These data emphasize the need for a well-thought-out extubation plan, with consideration of extubation when the patient is totally awake, during use of low-dose remifentanil, or over a guide for reintubation, such as an airway exchange catheter, among other techniques [17–19]. The Difficult Airway Society has produced guidelines for tracheal extubation which provide a practical stepwise approach to extubation [18].

Conclusion

With adequate knowledge of the factors precipitating critical incidents, injuries from these situations can be avoided. Searching for root causes of critical incidents and shedding light on the interactions among contributing factors that lead to them are necessary for developing effective prevention strategies and improving patient safety.

References

1. Kohn LT, Corrigan JM, Donaldson MS. To err is human: building a safer health system. Washington, DC: National Academy Press; 2000.
2. Lanier WL. A three-decade perspective on anesthesia safety. Am Surg. 2006;72(11):985–9.
3. Cooper JB, Newbower RS, Long CD, McPeek B. Preventable anesthesia mishaps: a study of human factors. Anesthesiology. 1978;49(6):399–406.
4. Vincent C. Understanding and responding to adverse events. N Engl J Med. 2003;348(11): 1051–6.
5. Dutton RP, DuKatz A. Quality improvement using automated data sources: the Anesthesia Quality Institute. Anesthesiol Clin. 2011;29(3):439–54.
6. Metzner J, Posner KL, Lam MS, Domino KB. Closed claims' analysis. Best Pract Res Clin Anaesthesiol. 2011;25(2):263–76.
7. Cheney FW. The American Society of Anesthesiologists Closed Claims Project: what have we learned, how has it affected practice, and how will it affect practice in the future? Anesthesiology. 1999;91(2):552–6.
8. Mehta SP, Bhananker SM, Posner KL, Domino KB. Operating room fires: a closed claims analysis. Anesthesiology. 2013;118(5):1133–9.
9. Greene BA. The hazard of fire and explosion in anesthesia: report of clinical investigation of 230 cases. Anesthesiology. 1941;2:141–60.
10. Greene BA. Hazards of fire and explosion of anesthetic agents. III. In presence of diathermy. Surg Gynecol Obstet. 1942;74:895–900.
11. Apfelbaum JL, Caplan RA, Barker SJ, Connis RT, Cowles C, Ehrenwerth J, et al. Practice advisory for the prevention and management of operating room fires: an updated report by the American Society of Anesthesiologists Task Force on Operating Room Fires. Anesthesiology. 2013;118(2):271–90.
12. Ziewacz JE, Arriaga AF, Bader AM, Berry WR, Edmondson L, Wong JM, et al. Crisis checklists for the operating room: development and pilot testing. J Am Coll Surg. 2011;213:212–9.
13. Arriaga AF, Bader AM, Wong JM, Lipsitz SR, Berry WR, Ziewacz JE, et al. Simulation-based trial of surgical-crisis checklists. N Engl J Med. 2013;368:246–53.
14. Apfelbaum JL, Hagbeg CA, Caplan RA, Blitt CD, Connis RT, Nickinovich DG, et al. Practice guidelines for management of the difficult airway: an updated report by the American Society of Anesthesiologists Task Force on Management of the Difficult Airway. Anesthesiology. 2013;118(2):251–70.
15. American Society of Anesthesiologist. Practice guidelines for management of the difficult airway. A report by the American Society of Anesthesiologists Task Force on Management of the Difficult Airway. Anesthesiology. 1993;78(3):597–602.
16. Peterson GN, Domino KB, Caplan RA, Posner KL, Lee LA, Cheney FW. Management of the difficult airway: a closed claims analysis. Anesthesiology. 2005;103(1):33–9.
17. Cavallone LF, Vannucci A; American Society of Anesthesiologists Task Force on Management of the Difficult Airway. Extubation of the difficult airway and extubation failure. Anesth Analg. 2013;116(2):368–83.

18. Difficult Airway Society Extubation Guidelines Group; Popat M, Mitchell V, Dravid R, Patel A, Swampillai C, et al. Difficult Airway Society Guidelines for the management of tracheal extubation. Anaesthesia. 2012;67(3):318–40.
19. Heidegger T. Extubation of the difficult airway—an important but neglected topic. Anaesthesia. 2012;67(3):213–5.

Chapter 4
Residency Training

Daniel Katz and Alan Sim

A Brief History of Anesthesiology Training

Formal training in anesthesiology has come a long way since the ether dome at Massachusetts General Hospital [1]. In fact, prior to our inception as a specialty in 1941 [2] there was little opportunity for structured training. Often times the role of the anesthetist fell to the surgical resident, a circulating nurse, or even medical students, with mortality rates as high as 50 % [3]. The need for formal training in anesthesiology was readily apparent.

In reality, the call for standards in anesthetic training actually predated our formal inception as a specialty with a resolution approved by the Board of Directors of the Society of Anesthetists in 1937, "It is to the best interest of the medical public that departments of anesthesia in medical schools and hospitals shall be in charge of physicians who shall have direct supervision of teaching of this subject to undergraduates and graduates. These physicians shall have devoted a satisfactory time to the study of the specialty or shall have been certified as specialists in anesthesia by a recognized national Society of Anesthetists" [4]. Since that time there has been much development by the now called American Society of Anesthesiologists (ASA) in formal residency training, with programs developing throughout the United States [5].

More needed to be done, however, as there were still major inconsistencies between different schools and programs. As such, a series of survey-based studies was undertaken in the late 1950s/early 1960s to better determine how programs were training their trainees [5]. Based on the results of the survey study, completed in 1966, the president of the ASA at that time, John J. Bonica, presented the report and its findings on how anesthesiologists were trained in the United States [6].

D. Katz, M.D. (✉) • A. Sim, M.D.
Department of Anesthesiology, Icahn School of Medicine at Mount Sinai,
KCC 8th Floor, One Gustave L. Levy Place, New York, NY 10029, USA
e-mail: dkatz621@gmail.com

As a result, several committees were created that would report to the Society's Council on Education including committees for Medical School Residencies, Internships, Anesthesia Residencies, and Post Graduate Training. These committees would be charged with ensuring a proper educational environment for anesthesiologists. Although these committees were independently run by the ASA, it was the Accreditation Council for Graduate Medical Education (ACGME) that truly standardized the graduate medical experience for the field of anesthesiology [7].

The Accreditation Council for Graduate Medical Education

Formed in 1981, the ACGME is an amalgam of regulatory bodies whose responsibility is the accreditation of graduate medical education (GME) [7]. It is the largest private professional accrediting agency in the United States, responsible for over 9,200 residency programs [8]. The ACGME has 28 committees (one for each of the 26 specialties, one for transitional year programs, and one for institutional review) [9]. While accreditation of a residency program by the ACGME is voluntary, accreditation is required to receive funding from the Center for Medicare and Medicaid Services (CMS). Additionally, residents must graduate from accredited programs to be eligible to take specialty boards [10]. Accreditation is granted after an application process consisting of about eight steps [11] (see Table 4.1).

ACGME Institutional Requirements

Prior to program accreditation, institutional accreditation must take place. Depending on the specific institution this process may already be completed. Institutional requirements focus on four main areas: organizational responsibilities, responsibilities for residents, the graduate medical education committee (GMEC), and internal review [12]. It requires written statements that the institution will

Table 4.1 Eight-step application process for ACGME accreditation

Step	Requirement	Specific for anesthesiology?
1	Determine if institutional accreditation is necessary	N/A
2	Determine if subspecialty is dependent or independent	Dependent
3	Review institutional and specialty requirements	Specialty requirements present
4	Determine deadline for submission of application	No site visit required
5	Complete the application form	Specific form required
6	Submit the application to your institutions GMEC and DIO	N/A
7	Send completed GMEC form to the RC	N/A
8	Contact your RC staff	Specific personnel for anesthesiology present

provide resources to support GME, with its own administrative system consisting of a designated institutional officer (DIO) and a GMEC who will ensure that the governing institution has the means and capabilities of overseeing GME programs. Additionally, it requires the institution to provide house staff with an appropriate appointment letter explaining responsibilities of the resident as well as the institution and benefits provided including:

Resident responsibilities
Duration of appointment
Financial support
Conditions for reappointment
Grievance process
Professional liability insurance
Health and disability insurance
Leaves of absence
Duty hour obligations
Moonlighting
Counseling services
Participation in educational and professional activities
Safe educational and work environments

Program Personnel and Resident Appointments

The anchor of any residency training program is the program director. As put forth by the ACGME the program director has "authority and accountability for the operation of the program" [13]. He/she must have administrative and specialty expertise including current board certification in his/her field. The program director must have a medical license and have an appropriate medical staff appointment. All program directors must be approved by the institution's GMEC. The responsibilities of the program director are very broad, and include but are not limited to:

Oversight of the didactic education material for residents
Selection of program faculty
Ensure proper program evaluation
Monitor resident supervision
Prepare and submit all paperwork to the ACGME
Provide each resident with semiannual feedback
Ensure compliance with grievance and due process procedures
Implement policies and procedures consistent with program requirements (i.e., moonlighting)

In general, program directors should have an energetic personality and should be enthusiastic about resident education. The nature of this position is quite demanding, as the program director is held accountable to not only the department and the ACGME but the residents as well. As such, the average expectancy for a tenure of program director averages about 7 years [14]. Programs that have a higher turnover rate may be subject to additional inquiries [13]. Substantial resources exist to aid new and veteran program directors alike, including a "Virtual Handbook" which provides program directors with the most current information they may need for their program [15].

The program director should be supported by a robust faculty and program personnel. Faculty physicians must have board certification in their specialty or will undergo further scrutiny by the review committee at the ACGME [16]. They should also demonstrate a dedication to resident education, with a curriculum of sufficient breadth and depth. The time faculty spend teaching and supervising residents should be documented and reported. Additionally, any off-campus rotation site should have a local director accountable for resident education and supervision. It is also recommended that faculty be involved in scholastic pursuits, including projects for the professional development of themselves and their residents [16]. Worthy academic pursuits should include organized rounds or teaching rounds, journal clubs, conferences, as well as traditional research projects. Ideally, faculty should therefore have peer-reviewed funding, publications in peer-reviewed journals, publications or presentations at meetings, and participation in national committees or other professional organizations.

Selection of residents is performed at the discretion of the individual program and should comply with their policies and procedures. Resident applicants must all meet the ACGME institutional requirements as well [17]. The number of residents allowed in a program is determined by the ACGME, and program directors are not allowed to increase the number of spots in a program without prior approval. As stated prior, all resident hires require a signed appointment letter.

Educational Program Components: The Core Competencies

One of the goals of resident education is to obtain a mastery of domains outside of the direct clinical arena. While much of the litany of material we are expected to master has been standardized (i.e., physiology, pharmacology), the manner in which we are trained to practice as physicians is not (i.e., bedside manner, professionalism). It is for this reason that in 2002 the ACGME developed an initiative called the Outcome Project [7]. They identified the six core competencies which would henceforth be used by GME programs to evaluate their residents. Since that time many graduate educators enhanced their educational programs to meet the objectives of the Outcome Project [18]. These six core competencies are patient care, medical knowledge, practice-based learning and improvement, interpersonal and communication skills, professionalism, and systems-based practice. While the ACGME discusses these competencies at length, let us investigate the competencies as they pertain to anesthesiology.

At the forefront of the core competencies is patient care. A resident must be able to provide care that is "compassionate, appropriate, and effective for the treatment

Table 4.2 Resident minimum case requirements for graduation

Clinical case/procedure	Minimum required
Spinal	40
Epidural	40
Peripheral nerve blockade	40
Special situation complex: trauma/burns	20
Cardiac with or without CBP (majority must be with CBP)	20
Intrathoracic noncardiac	20
Major vascular (open or endovascular)	20
Vaginal delivery (normal or high risk)	40
Cesarean section (normal or high risk)	20
Pain consultation (acute pain, chronic pain, and/or cancer pain)	20
Intracerebral (endovascular or open, majority must be open)	20
Pediatric cases: each category inclusive of younger patients	
<3 Months	5
<3 Years	20
<12 Years	100

of health problems and the promotion of health" [19]. As the level of experience allows, residents must demonstrate their ability to care for patients. Early in training, residents should be expected to treat patients with common diagnoses and for uncomplicated procedures, for example, provide an anesthetic for a laparoscopic cholecystectomy in a healthy patient. As they progress in training they should demonstrate proficiency in performing complex procedures such as the placement of a pulmonary artery catheter. To ensure that the anesthesiologist can meet this competency upon graduation, minimum requirements of cases and subspecialty procedures were added to the core requirement. The minimum case required for graduation is found in Table 4.2.

Right behind patient care is medical knowledge. Residents are expected to obtain sufficient knowledge of "biomedical, clinical, epidemiological-behavioral sciences" and know how to apply this knowledge to patient care [20]. Acquisition of this knowledge should occur from multiple sources including direct clinical teaching rounds, a robust didactic schedule, participation in multidisciplinary conferences, specialty meetings, journal clubs, and independent learning. Specific for anesthesiology, resident education should encompass a variety of topics both in and outside of the clinical arena. Required didactic topics are included in Table 4.3. While there is no minimum number of lectures required, a regular schedule should exist such that by the time residents complete the program they have been exposed to all the necessary topics. Regular involvement of department faculty is required, and it is strongly encouraged that the program director be directly involved in providing lectures and the didactic schedule. Resident run lectures should also be encouraged, and have been shown to improve resident satisfaction [21]. In addition to traditional didactics, e-learning modules and teleconference type lectures have also been successfully utilized [22, 23]. A robust didactic schedule is not only required,

Table 4.3 Required didactic topics for resident education

Required didactic topics	Potential inclusive topics
Basic science	Physiology
	Pharmacology
	Anatomy
Clinical anesthesiology	Subspecialty discussion
	Procedure-based topics
	Clinical dilemmas
Practice management	OR management
	Types of practice
	Financial planning
	Billing
	Regulatory issues
Management of the geriatric patient	Postoperative cognitive dysfunction
	Postoperative delirium
	Management of the patient with multiple medical problems
	Physiologic changes of aging
Management of the ambulatory surgical patient	Management of postoperative nausea and vomiting
	The ambulatory patient with morbid obesity
	Productivity at the ambulatory surgical center

Table 4.4 The PDSA cycle

PDSA cycle	Summary of cycle steps
Plan	Plan a change aimed at improvement
Do	Carry out the change
Study	Study the results of the change and focus on what worked, what went wrong, and why
Act	Adopt, abandon, or run the change through the cycle again

but regular attendance to morning conferences has been correlated with increased written board scores [24].

At the core of the practice-based learning and improvement competency is a commitment to lifelong learning and quality improvement [25]. It involves utilizing skills in self-assessment and reflection with the goal of improving practice. One such tool developed by Dr. Edwards Deming, called the P-D-S-A cycle or Plan, Do, Study, Act cycle [26], has been utilized by several industries and medicine subspecialties with great success [27–29]. A summary of the PDSA cycle can be found in Table 4.4. These cycles can be applied to clinically based improvement projects (improving cardiac case set-up times), personally oriented projects (stress or time management projects), or even practice-based projects (introduction of new ASA guidelines into practice). Inherent in this competency is the use of Evidence-Based Medicine (EBM), as many of the EBM-related skills, such as appraising and assimilating evidence into practice, are directly in line with this competency. Additionally, residents are required to participate in quality improvement (QI) initiatives, which can include participation in M&M conferences, membership to a QI committee, or analysis of a specific practice outcome [30–32]. Lastly, resident teaching skills are included in this domain. Residents are expected to obtain proficiency in educating patients, students, residents, families, and other members of the healthcare team. The role of the resident educator is discussed later below.

Good interpersonal and communication skills are critical for the practicing anesthesiologist, and as such, this core competency is one of the most important. According to the ACGME, residents in anesthesiology programs must "demonstrate interpersonal and communication skills that result in the effective exchange of information" [33]. This includes communication with patients and their families of different socioeconomic and cultural backgrounds aimed at general patient care as well as specific tasks such as the taking of a history, obtaining consent, and informing patients of the anesthetic and postoperative care plans. Residents should also be trained in communicating effectively with other members of the healthcare team, which is critical in the operating room environment where as much as 30 % of procedure-specific information can be lost due to miscommunication [34]. These types of errors can have dire consequences [35]. It is advised by the ACGME that this training not just be "On-the-job," but that residents should have a structured curriculum around this topic. Two such validated curricula include both Relationship Express [36] and Team STEPPS [37]. Lastly, residents are expected to maintain a comprehensive, timely, and legible medical record.

Proficiency in professionalism can be broken down into three major components: commitment, adherence, and sensitivity [38]. Residents are expected to be committed to their patients, treating them with respect, compassion, and empathy. Residents should adhere to ethical guidelines and show respect for patient autonomy and privacy. Additionally residents are expected to show sensitivity to a patient's culture, gender, age, and/or disability. Since this competency is behavioral in nature, it is often demonstrated through other competency domains. Evaluation tools on professionalism exist and are usually in the form of 360 evaluations [39]. While it may seem difficult to teach professionalism, it may be integrated into other didactics and case discussions. It may also be taught using role play, simulation, or small case vignettes [38]. It is most likely best learned through example, which is why promoting professionalism within the teaching faculty is important, as it can effect outcomes [40].

Proficiency in systems-based practice is based on the realization that the anesthesiologist is but one part in not only a clinical care team but also within a layer of the healthcare system [41]. Residents are therefore expected to work within various healthcare delivery locations and systems as well as be able to coordinate patient care within anesthesiology. Residents should be mindful of the costs of their interventions and should conduct risk–benefit analysis based on each patient. Within this core competency lies the expectation that the resident will work as part of an interprofessional and multidisciplinary team. For example, the anesthesiology resident is expected to work with not just his surgical and nursing colleagues, but must be proficient in coordinating care with patient floors, intensive care units, and other remote locations such as radiology and the labor and delivery floor. Our unique omnipresence in the hospital also makes us ideal candidates to identify system errors, and residents are expected to participate in the identification of these system errors as well as the implementation of solutions.

Anesthesiology residents are also required to participate in a yearly simulation activity as per this competency.

Program Design: Basic Requirements for the Clinical Base Year

According to the ACGME a minimum of 4 years of GME is required [42]. Of those 4 years, three must be dedicated to clinical anesthesiology (CA-1, CA-2, CA-3) with 1 clinical base year (CBY). The ACGME offers three options for anesthesiology-accredited programs. A program can offer a 3-year advanced track, a 4-year comprehensive track (including CBY), or a combination of the two options. Should the program opt for a 3-year advanced track prospective residents are required to match their CBY independent of their advanced program. Those residents have a choice of participating in a transitional, preliminary medicine, or preliminary surgical CBY. It is highly suggested that the CBY be completed before the resident begins CA-2 year, and it must be completed prior to beginning the CA-3 year. There are some advantages from the resident prospective in matching in a 1+3-year program. First, they will get clinical experience at another institution, which broadens their clinical experience. Second, it gives the resident flexibility of being in different locations for their training. Finally, the resident has more flexibility in the type of CBY, as he/she may choose from medicine, surgery, or a transitional curriculum. There are also advantages to the 4-year combined program. Residents of a 4-year program will only have to move once and may have a housing advantage over their 1+3 colleagues. Combined residents will also work within multiple departments of their home institution, which will make them familiar with the medical record and order entry systems, as well as the basic logistic layout of the institution. Additionally, interns of 4-year programs will be working side by side with their colleagues from other specialties, allowing them to form bonds with residents that they will be working with for the rest of their residency. Likewise, residents who pursue elective rotations in anesthesiology such as pain management are more likely to get credit toward their overall requirements since they will rotate through their respective parent department.

Regardless of the program chosen the requirements for the CBY are the same. In general, the resident should expect 12 months of broad education in various medical disciplines. They should be expected to be directly involved in decision making and should be responsible for patient care with adequate supervision. By the end of the year the resident should have basic fundamental competencies such as obtaining a complete medical history, performing a physical exam, basic patient assessment, and order appropriate diagnostic studies, and enact a treatment plan for a patient [42]. Specifically, residents must spend at least 6 months taking care of inpatients in internal medicine, pediatrics, surgery or surgical subspecialties, obstetrics and gynecology, neurology, and/or family medicine. It is recommended but not required that the residents have a rotation in critical care and emergency medicine of one, but not more than 2 months duration. Residents may take up to a 1-month rotation in anesthesiology during the CBY. Each month in the year can count for only one requirement, even if it crosses disciplines (i.e., a rotation in the surgical ICU can count as either surgery or critical care).

Program Design: Clinical Anesthesia Years (CA-1, CA-2, CA-3)

The goal of the clinical anesthesia years is to provide residents with a comprehensive background and proficiency in all areas of anesthesiology including preoperative, intraoperative, and postoperative care. Residents should also be versatile in the treatment and management of critically ill patients as well as those with chronic and acute pain. Training should be progressive in its complexity, allowing the resident to manage more difficult patients and procedures with proper supervision. By the end of training the resident should be "sufficiently independent" in clinical decision making and patient care and can lead a perioperative care team [42]. Required rotations and their respective lengths are found in Table 4.5.

In addition to the basic rotations residents are also encouraged by the ACGME to rotate through additional subspecialties (no more than 6 months) as well as other focused educational experiences [42]. For example, a resident interested in pediatric anesthesiology may choose to take rotations in the neonatal ICU, or rotate with a genetics expert, a pediatric infectious disease specialist, or a pediatric surgeon. Likewise, those interested in pain may pursue elective rotations in other related fields such as psychiatry, physical medicine and rehabilitation, and/or neurology. It is up to the discretion of the program director to allow residents to pursue these opportunities and weigh their educational and clinical merit. Residents may also request rotations at off-site locations, so long as there is adequate supervision, resources, a responsible local site director, and safe transport to the location.

Table 4.5 Required rotations for graduation

Rotation	Length
Obstetric anesthesia	Two 1-month rotations
Pediatric anesthesia	Two 1-month rotations
Neuroanesthesia	Two 1-month rotations
Cardiothoracic anesthesia	Two 1-month rotations
Critical care	Four distinct and progressive clinical months
Pain management	Three 1-month rotations
Preoperative evaluation	One-month rotation
PACU	0.5-month rotation

Note 2 months of critical care and 1 month of pain management can occur during the CBY

Resident Milestones and Examinations

Although residents are expected to progress linearly though their training, this is often not the case as not all residents are created equal. It is therefore prudent for the program director to set clinical and educational milestones that residents are expected to achieve. This is not done in a make or break manner, but serves as a tool to alert the program director that a resident may need remediation in a certain area. A basic milestone scheme is shown in Table 4.6.

In addition to clinical-based milestones, residents are expected to excel academically on standardized exams. The first series of examinations is referred to as the Anesthesia Knowledge Test or AKT. It is designed and distributed through a collaborative effort between Metrics and the Inter-Hospital Study Group for Anesthesia Education (IHSGAE) [43]. Residents in anesthesiology programs take three versions of the AKT at predetermined intervals. The first version of the test called the AKT-1 is taken twice. It is taken on the first day of anesthesiology residency (CA-1 year) and then taken again at day 30. This first test is not a metric for the residents, but is in fact a measure of a program's ability to teach their residents a basic knowledge of anesthesia [44]. It focuses on the basics of cardiopulmonary resuscitation and the knowledge needed to administer an anesthetic to a healthy, uncomplicated patient presenting for simple surgery. The second AKT is the AKT-6, taken 6 months into CA-1 year, and is made up of eight major areas including anesthesia, cardiovascular, equipment, neuromuscular, pharmacology, regional anesthesia and pain therapy, respiration, and miscellaneous. Like the AKT-1 it is used to evaluate both resident progression and program adequacy. The last AKT, the AKT-24, is taken at the end of CA-2 year. It is designed specifically to test the subspecialty knowledge of the CA-2 resident in seven areas including perioperative medicine, critical care, cardiovascular, neuroanesthesia, pain management, pediatrics, and obstetrics. Examinees are asked to mark on their score sheet which subspecialties they have rotated through for comparative purposes [44].

Every year on the first Saturday in March residents will also take the in-training examination administered by the American Board of Anesthesiology (ABA). It is a 4 h long voluntary computer-based test. The contents of the exam are the same regardless of the clinical year (each resident has a test made from the same pool

Table 4.6 Example resident milestones

Time period	Resident milestone
0–1 Months	The resident is able to be left alone for very brief periods (less than 5 min) in uncomplicated cases with stable patients
1–3 Months	The resident is able to be double covered for simple cases
6 Months	The resident is capable to be a first responder to simple floor intubations with immediate back-up available
10–13 Months	The resident has demonstrated the ability to begin subspecialty rotations
24 Months	The resident has demonstrated the ability to lead a perioperative care team
36 Months	The resident has demonstrated the ability to practice independently

of questions), in contrast to the AKT. Residents in 4-year categorical program are often expected to take the in-training examination during their CBY, while residents who are in preliminary years may not have this opportunity. The examination covers every area relevant to anesthesiology including basic science, clinical science, organ-based basic and clinical sciences, clinical subspecialties, as well as special problems or issues in anesthesiology [45].

Besides the AKT and in-training exam, residents who will complete training after June 30, 2016, will also take a staged version of the written boards (Part 1 Examination) at the beginning of their CA-2 year (July 2014) [46]. This examination, now called the BASIC examination, will focus on basic content areas such as pharmacology, physiology, anatomy, anesthesia equipment, and monitoring. The ADVANCED exam will still be administered after graduation from an ACGME-accredited program and will focus on subspecialty areas, but will also cover all topics present in the BASIC exam.

Resident Requirements: ACGME Duty Hours, Logs, and Evaluations

The death of Libby Zion at the hands of a resident in a New York Hospital in 1984 sparked great interest in limiting duty hours for house staff [47]. In New York State, the Libby Zion law, also known as the Bell Commission, was passed in 1989 limiting residents to work no more than 80 h/week and for no more than 24 h in a row [48]. At that time these restrictions were met with much resistance, as programs claimed that restricting hours was detrimental to training competent physicians and that programs would have to increase residency times to compensate. In fact, it was believed that several institutions ignored these rules outright, especially those outside of New York [47].

However, in 2003 the ACGME released their own mandatory work hour restrictions, which looked very similar to the standards set by the Bell Commission [49]. Now programs would have to comply with the work hour restrictions or risk losing accreditation. Since that time there have been many revisions and expansions to work hour rules, aimed at preventing resident fatigue and improving patient care. Additionally, programs are now required to have didactic sessions on resident fatigue, stress management, and sleep deprivation [42]. Concerns about increased errors by increasing the amount of patient handoffs exist, and multiple specialties have expressed concerns that these new duty hour restrictions either negatively affect their programs or are ineffective in decreasing errors and resident fatigue [50–52]. A summary of the ACGME duty hour rules is found in Table 4.7.

To ensure compliance with duty hour regulations residents are required to maintain accurate logs of their duty hours. It is recommended the hours be entered daily to increase accuracy, but it is not required. These logs are regularly reviewed by both the program director and the GMEC of the institution. Multiple logging systems exist; however, many institutions have adopted systems such as New Innovations

Table 4.7 ACGME duty hours summary [42]

ACGME rule	Interpretation	Exceptions/caveats
80 h rule	Duty hours must be limited to 80 h/week averaged over a 1-month period	Final year residents can extend their week to provide continuity of care of critical importance and unique educational value to the resident
Mandatory time free of duty	One duty free day every week (averaged over 4 weeks) is required	None, home call may not be assigned on free days
Maximum duty period length	PGY-1 residents: 16 h	For PGY-2 residents, napping between 10 p.m. and 8 a.m. after 16 h of duty is suggested
	PGY-2 residents: 24 h	Residents are allowed 4 h of nonclinical duty time for transition of care after a 24 h shift
Minimum time off between duty periods	PGY-1 and intermediate residents should have 10 h, must have 8 h off between shifts	Final year residents may have less than 8 h off between shifts at the discretion of the program director so long as the extra duty time is of high educational value
	PGY-2 residents must have 14 h off after a 24 h shift	
Maximum in-house night float	No more than six consecutive nights	
Maximum in-house on-call frequency	PGY-2 and above may be scheduled for no more than every third night (over a 4-week period)	
At-home call	Time spent in hospital counts toward 80 h maximum	May be more frequent than every third night but must not preclude reasonable amounts of rest and personal time for residents
Moonlighting	All moonlighting shifts count toward duty hours and must remain compliant	
	PGY-1 residents may not moonlight	

which allow residents to view and edit their duty hour logs. These systems allow residents to input the type of duty hours worked (Home Call vs. In House Call vs. OR Shifts, etc.) and will automatically alert them to work hour violations. Residents may also enter their vacations into the system.

Anesthesiology residents are also required to keep a log of their cases and procedures. This data may be entered into the ACGME's Resident Case Log System [53]. The data entered into this system is encrypted and is used by the ACGME for accreditation purposes only [54]. Residents can track their case logs in real time, and compare the cases entered against a template with required minimum cases to alert residents who may be deficient in certain clinical areas. Additional fields are provided as descriptors for procedures that are encouraged but not required (i.e., using ultrasound for a peripheral nerve block). No patient identifiable information should be entered into this log.

In addition to case and duty hour logs, residents and faculty are also required to complete evaluations. Formal evaluations must be completed in a timely manner during each rotation. As per the ACGME, for each rotation the program must provide objective assessments of the resident in relation to the core competencies, use multiple evaluators (faculty, peers, patients, etc.), document progressive resident performance, and provide each resident with documented evaluations on a semiannual basis. These evaluations must be accessible by the resident for review [42]. Additionally, upon completion of residency the program director must also provide a summative evaluation of the resident to be placed into the permanent record. This evaluation must also be accessible to the resident and must document resident performance and verify competence sufficient to enter practice [55]. Likewise, the program must also evaluate faculty on an annual basis, which should include reviews of the faculty member's teaching ability, commitment to education, clinical knowledge, professionalism, and scholarly activities. Faculty evaluations must include written confidential evaluations by residents [42]. To complete the circle, the program must also evaluate itself. It must monitor and track progress at least annually in the following areas: resident performance, graduate performance (performance on certification examinations), faculty development, and program quality. Both residents and faculty must participate confidentially and in writing to this evaluation at least annually [42]. If the program is found to be inadequate in any area the program must create a formal written action plan. Specifically for anesthesiology, the ACGME also obtains data from the ABA on the most recent board examination scores. At least 70 % of residents should be certified in the latest 5-year period [42]. Several modes of evaluation exist from web surveys, to paper forms; however, many programs utilize standardized surveys from companies such as New Innovations [56] or MyEvaluations [57] to ensure quality and anonymity. If any resident believes their evaluations are not anonymous, they can report their concerns to their local GMEC, their departmental ombudsperson, or to the ACGME directly.

The New Anesthesiology Resident: Clinician, Researcher, Clinical Educator

As one can see, the role of the resident is dynamic and growing. Whereas in the past residents in anesthesiology were focused on clinical competence, resident responsibilities have expanded. Residents are now given specific goals and objectives which must be met on their clinical rotations as well as demonstrate proficiency in the core competencies, increasing in complexity as training progresses. Standardized exams are increasing in number as well, ensuring that residents are up to date on their education. Clinical duties have also expanded, requiring anesthesiology residents to not only be proficient in the OR but also be able to practice as leaders of perioperative teams and perioperative consulting physicians, able to practice in a variety of clinical environments.

Participation in scholarly activity is also required, including proficiency in the basic principles of research. Each resident must complete an academic assignment, usually during CA-2 or CA-3 years which may include presentations at grand rounds, publications in journals, authorship of book chapters, or clinical instruction manuals [42]. In fact, programs that have structured educational curricula have benefitted from this requirement, seeing increased amounts of research productivity from their residents [58].

Finally, now more than ever, anesthesiology residents are expected to be clinical educators to their peers, medical students, patients and their families, as well as other healthcare professionals [42]. After all, the term "doctor" is taken from the Latin word "docere," which means "to teach" [59]. While formal education-based curricula existed as early as the 1970s [60], by 2001, about half of all residency programs in the United States offered formal training in educational and teaching skills [61]. Programs around the country are now offering clinical education fellowship position or integrated clinical educator tracks [62], allowing residents to be not only first rate clinicians but first rate educators as well.

References

1. Fenster JM. Ether day: the strange tale of America's greatest medical discovery and the haunted men who made it. New York: Harper Collins; 2001.
2. Betcher AM, Ciliberti BJ, Wood PM, Wright LH. The jubilee year of organized anesthesia. Anesthesiology. 1956;17:266.
3. Larson MD. History of anesthetic practice [Internet]. Miller's anesthesia. 7th ed. Amsterdam: Elsevier; 1846. p. 1–41. Available from: http://dx.doi.org/10.1016/B978-0-443-06959-8.00001-7
4. Meeting A 9th. Collected papers and minutes of the Long Island, New York and American Society of Anesthetists (1905–1936); 1936. p. Volume I.
5. Albert M. Betcher M. The Genesis of Contemporary American Anesthesiology. Volpitto, Vandam LD; 1982. p. 185–121.
6. Handbook for Delegates. The American Society of Anesthesiologists. Annual Meeting; 1965.
7. Taradejna C. ACGME history [Internet]. 2007. Available from: http://www.acgme.org/acgmeweb/About/ACGMEHistory.aspx
8. About ACGME [Internet]. 2013. Available from: http://www.acgme.org/acgmeweb/tabid/116/About.aspx
9. ACGME at a Glance [Internet]. 2013. Available from: http://www.acgme.org/acgmeweb/About/ACGMEataGlance.aspx
10. ACGME Fact Sheet [Internet]. 2013. Available from: http://www.acgme.org/acgmeweb/About/Newsroom/FactSheet.aspx
11. ACGME How to Apply for Accreditation in Eight Steps. 2013;(c):2–9 Available from: http://dconnect.acgme.org/acgmeweb/Portals/0/application-process-eight-easy-steps.pdf
12. Directors FP. ACGME Institutional Requirements. p. 1–4.
13. Program, Personnel, and Resources: Program Director. 2008;(1):5–7. Available from: http://acgme.org/acgmeweb/Portals/0/PDFs/commonguide/IIA_ProgramDirector_Explanation.pdf
14. Analysis D of O and D. Average length in years between program director appointment dates; 2007.
15. Program Director's "Virtual Handbook" [Internet]. 2013. Available from: http://www.acgme.org/acgmeweb/tabid/279/GraduateMedicalEducation/InstitutionalReview/ProgramDirectorsVirtualHandbook.aspx
16. II. Program Personnel and Resources B. Faculty and C. Other program personnel common program requirement. 2008. Available from: http://acgme.org/acgmeweb/Portals/0/PDFs/commonguide/IIBC_FacultyandOtherProgramPersonnel_Explanation.pdf
17. Resident Appointments; 2008.

18. Swing SR. The ACGME outcome project: retrospective and prospective. Med Teach. 2007; 29(7):648–54. Available from: http://www.ncbi.nlm.nih.gov/pubmed/18236251
19. Patient Care [Internet]. 2008. p. 2008. Available from: http://acgme.org/acgmeweb/Portals/0/PDFs/commonguide/IVA5a_EducationalProgram_ACGMECompetencies_PatientCare_Explanation.pdf
20. Medical Knowledge [Internet]. 2008. p. 2008. Available from: http://acgme.org/acgmeweb/Portals/0/PDFs/commonguide/IVA5b_EducationalProgram_ACGMECompetencies_MedicalKnowledge_Explanation.pdf
21. Farrohki ET, Jensen AR, Brock DM, Cole JK, Mann GN, Pellegrini CA, et al. Expanding resident conferences while tailoring them to level of training: a longitudinal study. J Surg Educ. 2008;65(2):84–90. Available from: http://www.ncbi.nlm.nih.gov/pubmed/18439525
22. Markova, T., Roth L. E-conferencing for Delivery of Residency Didactics. Acad Med 2002;77(7):748-9
23. Sajeva M. E-learning: Web-based education. Curr Opin Anaesthesiol. 2006;19(6):645–9. Available from: http://www.ncbi.nlm.nih.gov/pubmed/17093369
24. Landers DF, Becker GL, Newland MC, Peters KR. Lecture practices in United States anesthesiology residencies. Anesth Analg. 1992;74(1):112–5. Available from: http://www.ncbi.nlm.nih.gov/pubmed/1734770
25. Practice-based Learning and Improvement [Internet]. 2009. p. 8–9. Available from: http://acgme.org/acgmeweb/Portals/0/PDFs/commonguide/IVA5c_EducationalProgram_ACGMECompetencies_PBLI_Explanation.pdf
26. Moen R, Norman C. Evolution of the PDCA Cycle. 1–11. Available from: http://pkpinc.com/files/NA01MoenNormanFullpaper.pdf
27. Anderson C. How are PDCA cycles used. Bizmanualz [Internet]. June 2011. Available from: http://www.bizmanualz.com/blog/how-are-pdca-cycles-used-inside-iso-9001.html
28. Curran ET, Bunyan D. Using a PDSA cycle of improvement to increase preparedness for, and management of, norovirus in NHS Scotland. J Hosp Infect. 2012;82(2):108–13. Available from: http://www.ncbi.nlm.nih.gov/pubmed/22944362
29. Michael M, Schaffer SD, Egan PL, Little BB, Pritchard PS. Improving wait times and patient satisfaction in primary care. J Healthc Qual. 2013;35(2):50–9; quiz 59–60. Available from: http://www.ncbi.nlm.nih.gov/pubmed/23480405
30. Falcone JL, Lee KKW, Billiar TR, Hamad GG. Practice-based learning and improvement: a two-year experience with the reporting of morbidity and mortality cases by general surgery residents. J Surg Educ. 2012;69(3):385–92. Available from: http://www.ncbi.nlm.nih.gov/pubmed/22483142
31. Thomas MK, McDonald RJ, Foley EF, Weber SM. Educational value of morbidity and mortality (M&M) conferences: are minor complications important? J Surg Educ. 2012;69(3):326–9. Available from: http://www.ncbi.nlm.nih.gov/pubmed/22483132
32. Bevis KS, Straughn JM, Kendrick JE, Walsh-Covarrubias J, Kilgore LC. Morbidity and mortality conference in obstetrics and gynecology: a tool for addressing the 6 core competencies. J Grad Med Educ. 2011;3(1):100–3. Available from: http://www.pubmedcentral.nih.gov/articlerender.fcgi?artid=3186274&tool=pmcentrez&rendertype=abstract
33. Interpersonal and Communication Skills [Internet]. 2008. p. 2008. Available from: http://acgme.org/acgmeweb/Portals/0/PDFs/commonguide/IVA5d_EducationalProgram_ACGMECompetencies_IPCS_Explanation.pdf
34. Gillespie BM, Chaboyer W, Fairweather N. Interruptions and miscommunications in surgery: an observational study. AORN J. 2012;95(5):576–90. Available from: http://www.ncbi.nlm.nih.gov/pubmed/22541769
35. Neily J, Mills PD, Eldridge N, Dunn EJ, Samples C, Turner JR, et al. Incorrect surgical procedures within and outside of the operating room. Arch Surg. 2009;144(11):1028–34. Available from: http://www.ncbi.nlm.nih.gov/pubmed/19917939
36. Berger JS, Blatt B, McGrath B, Greenberg L, Berrigan MJ. Relationship express: a pilot program to teach anesthesiology residents communication skills. J Grad Med Educ. 2010;2(4):600–3. Available from: http://www.pubmedcentral.nih.gov/articlerender.fcgi?artid=3010947&tool=pmcentrez&rendertype=abstract

37. Team Stepps [Internet]. 2013. Available from: http://teamstepps.ahrq.gov/
38. Professionalism [Internet]. 2008. p. 5–6. Available from: http://acgme.org/acgmeweb/Portals/0/PDFs/commonguide/IVA5e_EducationalProgram_ACGMECompetencies_Professionalism_Explanation.pdf
39. Meng L, Metro D. Evaluating professionalism and interpersonal and communication skills: implementing a 360-degree evaluation instrument in an Anesthesiology Residency Program. J Grad Med Educ. 2009;1(2):216–20.
40. Bahaziq W, Crosby E. Physician professional behaviour affects outcomes: a framework for teaching professionalism during anesthesia residency. Can J Anaesth. 2011;58(11):1039–50. Available from: http://www.ncbi.nlm.nih.gov/pubmed/21866428
41. Systems Based Practice [Internet]. 2008. Available from: http://acgme.org/acgmeweb/Portals/0/PDFs/commonguide/IVA5f_EducationalProgram_ACGMECompetencies_SBP_Explanation.pdf
42. ACGME Program Requirements [Internet]. 2008. p. 1–31. Available from: http://www.acgme.org/acgmeweb/Portals/0/PFAssets/ProgramRequirements/040_anesthesiology_f07012011.pdf
43. Metrics [Internet]. Available from: http://www.metricsinc.org/
44. The Interhospital Group for Anesthesia Education [Internet]. Available from: http://www.metricsinc.org/ihsgae.htm
45. ABA. In-training content outline [Internet]. Available from: http://www.theaba.org/pdf/ITEContentOutline.pdf
46. ABA. Staged examinations [Internet]. Available from: http://www.theaba.org/Home/TrainingPrograms
47. Lerner B. A life-changing case for doctors in training. New York Times [Internet]. New York; 3 March 2009. Available from: http://www.nytimes.com/2009/03/03/health/03zion.html?_r=0
48. Lerner B. A case that shook medicine. The Washington Post [Internet]. Washington, DC; 28 Nov 2006. Available from: http://www.washingtonpost.com/wp-dyn/content/article/2006/11/24/AR2006112400985.html
49. Philibert I, Friedmann P, Williams WT. New requirements for resident duty hours. JAMA. 2002;288(9):1112–4. Available from: http://www.ncbi.nlm.nih.gov/pubmed/12204081
50. Roehr B. Reducing interns' duty hours is problematic, studies show. BMJ. 2013;346:f1998. Available from: http://www.bmj.com/cgi/doi/10.1136/bmj.f1998
51. Desai S V, Feldman L, Brown L, Dezube R, Yeh H-C, Punjabi N, et al. Effect of the 2011 vs 2003 duty hour regulation-compliant models on sleep duration, trainee education, and continuity of patient care among internal medicine house staff: a randomized trial. JAMA. 2013;173(8):649–55. Available from: http://www.ncbi.nlm.nih.gov/pubmed/23529771
52. Drolet BC, Sangisetty S, Tracy TF, Cioffi WG. Surgical residents' perceptions of 2011 accreditation council for graduate medical education duty hour regulations. JAMA. 2013;148(5):427–33. Available from: http://www.ncbi.nlm.nih.gov/pubmed/23677406
53. ACGME Case Log System [Internet]. 2013. Available from: https://www.acgme.org/connect/login?ReturnUrl=%2fconnect%2fissue%2fwsfed%3fwa%3dwsignin1.0%26wtrealm%3dhttps%253a%252f%252fwww.acgme.org%252fResidentDataCollectionNet%252fACGME%252fResidentCaselogs%252fCaselogsHome.aspx%26wctx%3drm%253d0%2526id%253dpassive%2526ru%253d%25252fResidentDataCollectionNet%25252fACGME%25252fResidentCaseLogs%25252fLogin.aspx%26wct%3d2013-05-27T21%253a58%253a30Z%26whr%3dacgme-us
54. ACGME. Resident case log system [Internet]. Available from: http://www.acgme.org/acgmeweb/DataCollectionSystems/ResidentCaseLogSystem.aspx
55. Common Program Requirements; 2011. p. 1–19.
56. New Innovations, INC. [Internet]. 2013. Available from: http://www.new-innov.com/pub/rms/main.aspx
57. Evaluations M. MyEvaluations.com [Internet]. 2013. Available from: https://www.myevaluations.com/
58. Ahmad S, De Oliveira GS, McCarthy RJ. Status of anesthesiology resident research education in the United States: structured education programs increase resident research productivity. Anesth Analg. 2013;116(1):205–10. Available from: http://www.ncbi.nlm.nih.gov/pubmed/23223116

59. The Latin Dictionary [Internet]. 2013. Available from: http://latindictionary.wikidot.com/verb:docere
60. Meleca C. A house staff training program to improve clinical teaching. Conf Res Med Educ. 1977;16:332–3.
61. Morrison EH, Friedland JA, Boker J, Rucker L, Hollingshead JMP. Residents as teachers training in U.S. residency programs and offices of graduate medical education. Acad Med. 2001;76:S1–4.
62. A L. Program Overview [Internet]. 2013. Available from: http://icahn.mssm.edu/departments-and-institutes/anesthesiology/programs-and-services/anesthesiology-residency

Chapter 5
Requirements for a Fellowship

Sarah AbdelFattah and William Peruzzi

Education in Anesthesiology Fellowship Training

During anesthesiology training, there comes a point where a critical decision must be made, i.e., private practice vs. academia, fellowship or no fellowship, and location of training and practice. The purpose of this chapter is to aid in the understanding of the different fellowships available, the requirements for each, and what advantages the additional training may yield.

Expectations of doing a fellowship may vary depending on which fellowship is chosen as well as the motivation of the resident involved. A fellowship allows for future personal fulfillment within a given scope of anesthesia [1]. Although most people will decide whether or not to complete more training, the physician will base the decision on economics and/or timing, as it inherently comes down to value. The value of further educating oneself not only will pay off financially over years to come, but it also will give one some separation and a distinct quality of skills that will be sought after. Fellowships allow physicians to gain more perspective within a field and give opinions based on that knowledge acquired within that time frame. This acquired skill set will help with making better healthcare decisions, allow one to gain more confidence in those decisions, as well as help in job security in the field of anesthesia.

There are several fellowships that can be pursued after doing an anesthesiology residency. They fall into one of three categories: (1) accredited fellowships with board certification examination, (2) accredited fellowships without board examination, and (3) non-accredited fellowships.

S. AbdelFattah, M.D. • W. Peruzzi, M.D., S.M., F.C.C.M. (✉)
Department of Anesthesiology, Perioperative Medicine & Pain Management,
Jackson Memorial Hospital, University of Miami, Miller School of Medicine,
1611 NW 12th Avenue (C-301), Miami, FL 33136, USA
e-mail: WPeruzzi@med.miami.edu

Accredited Fellowships with Board Certification Examinations

Several subspecialties offer fellowships, some with additional certification.

Critical Care Medicine

The subspecialty of Critical Care Medicine (CCM) in anesthesiology focuses on the care, both short and long term, of patients with significant organ system dysfunction [2]. This may encompass serious derangements in a single organ system or varying degrees of dysfunction in multiple organ systems. Because of the inherent nature of critical illnesses, end-of-life and palliative care experiences are also an integral part of the learning process.

ACGME-accredited CCM fellowships are generally 12 months in duration, although they may be longer if significant research components are incorporated. During the training period, at least 9 of the 12 months must be in the care of critically ill patients and preferably organized in such a fashion so as to provide a multispecialty (i.e., surgical, medical, neurologic) experience. There is a requirement that some pediatric training be incorporated into adult training programs, but the means by which to accomplish this education are often left to the discretion of the program directors and may include didactics as well as direct clinical experiences. It is expected that patient census of intensive care units (ICUs) within which training takes place will have an average census of at least five patients [2].

The remaining 3 months of "elective" training may be outside of the critical care environment but related to the specialty. Some programs dedicate this time to research, echocardiography, or related areas such as transfusion medicine, palliative care, radiology, or hyperbaric medicine.

In addition to the multispecialty focus of CCM training, there should be an emphasis on multidisciplinary education that includes clinical pharmacists, dieticians, physical and occupational therapists, speech-language pathologists, nursing, and respiratory care comprise the team needed to support and encourage the healing and recovery process of the high-acuity critically ill patient population.

An anesthesiology-based CCM fellowship program can only exist in an institution with an ACGME-accredited anesthesiology residency or in an institution with a formal integration agreement with the core training program. The program director must be board certified in the specialty and must be a medical director or co-medical director of the critical care unit(s) in which the majority of fellowship training takes place and must be personally involved in clinical supervision and teaching within that unit(s).

The faculty complement must have proper skills and qualifications to supervise the CCM fellows, and the ratio of anesthesiology CCM faculty to fellows can be no less than 1:2 [2]. The multispecialty and multidisciplinary nature of CCM lends itself to collaboration with others in various clinical arenas. Regular multidisciplinary rounds on patients not only improve patient care but provide an opportunity for exchange of ideas regarding clinical and basic research, technology adoption or development, process improvement efforts, and much more.

Aside from the broad clinical experience needed to become an accomplished intensivist, the successful CCM fellowship provides an opportunity for the fellows to become the consummate consultant. An intensivist must be capable of coordinating care amongst multiple clinical subspecialists and setting therapeutic priorities based on the overall needs of the patient ("the forest"), rather than the individual focus of each person involved ("the trees"). This skill is really best described as crew resource management (CRM) which focuses on the most effective utilization of skills and resources plus development of effective communications systems, situational awareness, decision making, problem solving, and teamwork.

Pain Medicine

The pain fellowship in anesthesiology, like CCM, is a 12-month program that has similar curricula offered through several other primary specialties including neurology, internal medicine, physical medicine and rehabilitation, and some psychiatry training programs. The application process in anesthesiology involves a match program similar to the transition from medical school to residency [3]. Only multidisciplinary programs are accredited and only in institutions that also sponsor residencies in at least two of the four potential residency programs (anesthesiology, neurology, physical medicine and rehabilitation, or psychiatry) [1]. This process permits fellows to often work closely with faculty and co-fellows that have trained in residencies outside of their own. In addition to providing differing perspectives in the treatment of pain, the system allows for the development of teamwork practices that are so very important to the successful management of these patients.

Fellows may expect to have a curriculum designed to provide them with the knowledge and skills to be facile and autonomous with multimodal pain management. Such an educational plan should involve experience in multiple clinical scenarios including acute pain management, neuropathic pain syndromes, cancer-related pain, and palliative care [4]. There should be a wide gamut of pain problems available for assessment and treatment. The clinical experience must provide for continuity of care experience (inpatient to outpatient), especially as it relates to cancer pain management and palliative care. The resources needed for proper pain management training must include adequate imaging facilities, psychiatric/psychological/behavioral services, social services, and electrodiagnostics. Focus on enteral as well as intravenous medications and management of patients using the World Health Organization (WHO) ladder a learning goal. The clinical skill of recognizing when intervention outside of these medications is needed will also be acquired.

Interventional pain training may include injections of the cervical, thoracic, and lumbar spine, injection of major joints, sympathetic blocks, spinal cord stimulation procedures, and placement of intrathecal drug delivery systems. Most of these procedures be performed in an outpatient or ambulatory care setting, but proper monitoring facilities must be present wherever the procedure is performed. Fellows learn to perform procedures on the basis of anatomical landmarks, with real-time fluoroscopic guidance and other technology, as appropriate.

Accredited Fellowships Without Board Certification Examinations

Cardiothoracic Anesthesiology

Cardiothoracic anesthesia is an accredited ACGME recognized fellowship [5]. The focus is on cardiac anesthesia as well as noncardiac cases. The curriculum usually involves didactic teaching on practice management, major cardiac cases, cardiac anesthesia outside the operating room, and management of cardiopulmonary bypass. There is also a focus on mechanical and assist devices such as LVADs (left ventricular assistive devices), RVADs (right ventricular assist devices), and other mechanical devices that are noninvasive. Education on Extracorporeal Membrane Oxygenation (ECMO) management can also be expected while working closely with surgical teams as well as perfusionists in caring for these patients [5].

Additionally, focus on management of congenital heart diseases intraoperatively and major intrathoracic vascular cases can be expected during the fellowship. One can also expect advanced transesophageal echocardiography (TEE)/transthoracic echocardiography (TTE) certification and eligibility to sit for the examination. Most fellows are eligible for advanced certification, depending on the number of examinations completed under attending supervision during the fellowship. There are many forms of certification. It is offered in (1) transthoracic two-dimensional and Doppler echocardiography interpretation, (2) transesophageal echocardiography, (3) transthoracic along with transesophageal echocardiography, (4) transthoracic with stress echocardiography, (5) a comprehensive certification which includes all of the preceding certifications, and finally (6) basic or advanced perioperative TEE. Most fellows in cardiothoracic anesthesia and some of those completing a critical care fellowship will be able to gain certification.

According to the National Board of Echocardiography, there are two pathways to gain certification. One pathway is termed the "experience requirement" where one can document a 12-month fellowship with experience taking care of perioperative surgical patients with cardiovascular disease. There should be 150 patients per year seen in the 2 years prior to application. The second pathway is called the "training pathway" which is where most physicians will fall under. This program includes 300 complete examinations within 4 years immediately prior to application [3]. Half of these exams can include those done by someone else but are interpreted by the person seeking certification. This training requires at least 50 h of American Medical Association category I continuing medical education focused on echocardiography. This along with a notarized letter from either a division director, director of cardiac anesthesiology, or an anesthesiology department chair will allow for certification [5].

The fellowship comprises a minimum of 12 months, beginning after completion of an anesthesia residency [1]. Fellows must be ACLS providers as well.

Starting in the 2014–2015 fellowship year, this fellowship will go through a match process. Applicants will register through the SF (San Francisco based matching program) and provide a rank list, just as was done for residency. There are a few exceptions that will apply during this match process, including applicants on military leave of absence, internal candidates who are currently training at the same institution where they want to do fellowship, applications to reside outside the United States at the time of application as well as those enrolled in anesthesiology residency at the time of application [5]. The applicants to which these exceptions may apply still need to register and partake in the ranking process but will fill out an exception agreement should it apply.

Pediatric Anesthesiology

Pediatric anesthesiology fellowship provide broad clinical knowledge in the approach to the care of neonates, infants, children, and adolescents in all surgical subspecialties [6]. Education is focused on the anatomical, physiological, as well as developmental and behavioral changes along the spectrum of ages throughout the early years of life. Fellows can expect certification in Pediatric and Neonatal Advanced Life Support (PALS) as well [6]. There is also a focus on technical skills needed for the delicate nature of children as well as management of difficult airways in children with congenital abnormalities.

The pediatric fellowship is another participant of the match program. This is done through the NRMP (National Resident Matching Program) site. Usually, the registration and interview process is in January through May of the year prior to the planned start of the fellowship year [1, 6]. Beginning in August and at the latest mid September, rank lists are submitted. Match day is usually in early October [3]. Most residents/applicants find positions through the match, but there is also a good portion that will find jobs outside the match. When this happens, those candidates, if they accept an offer outside the match, must withdraw from the match.

Starting in October 2013, there will be an annual Pediatric Anesthesiology Examination for all physicians interested in subspecialty certification in pediatric anesthesiology [6]. The test includes those physicians that are interested in qualification via "grandfathering," that is, those who have been practicing pediatric anesthesiology for a period of time after residency who never had an option for certification. According to the American Board of Anesthesiologists, no more than

7 years can have elapsed between a physician's completion of residency and board certification.

Non-accredited Fellowships

Obstetric Anesthesiology

Obstetric anesthesiology is a very well-defined discipline within anesthesiology devoted to the understanding of the perioperative management of the parturient [7]. Like most of the fellowships through anesthesiology, it composes of a minimum of 12 months [1]. Fellows in obstetric anesthesiology can expect to receive a comprehensive understanding of women during pregnancy and the puerperium as well as a wide variety of clinical scenarios that can occur in the pregnant state. The various risks involved with disease states that are specific to pregnancy, such as preeclampsia and eclampsia, as well as patients with chronic diseases that may be highlighted or exaggerated during pregnancy will be a learning objective. Additionally, neuraxial anesthesia in the form of epidural, intrathecal, and combined procedures as well as intravenous options and general anesthetics in this population will be proficiencies the fellow can expect. Fellows will become experts at the anesthesia and analgesia involved in spontaneous vaginal delivery, operative vaginal delivery, cesarean delivery, and emergent cesarean delivery in patients along the spectrum of health [7]. There will also be emphasis on understanding fetal heart rate measurement and interpretation.

Fellows will also become experts at the management of pregnant women going for non-pregnancy-related surgeries as well as surgeries necessary for the fetus while in utero. These may include less complicated cases such as intra-abdominal processes or orthopedic cases to more complicated cases, such as those involving fetoscopic surgery or those involving ex utero intrapartum treatment (EXIT) and need for ECMO (extracorporeal membrane oxygenation) for the neonate. Rotations may involve obstetric subspecialties involving intrauterine implantation of fertilized eggs reproductive endocrinology or those focused on patients with chronic diseases maternal-fetal medicine.

Neonatal resuscitation is also a learning objective within the fellowship year. This skill can be obtained via certification through the American Academy of Pediatrics Neonatal Resuscitation Program which is in association with the American Heart Association. This will provide necessary skills and information needed to aid in the newly born baby with respiratory distress or other life-challenging situations. These classes are usually divided over nine lessons along with five hands-on training exercises.

With our ever-aging population and disease states with longer life expectancies, one can expect to manage a multitude of disease states that will involve a multidisciplinary approach. This will result in a very well rounded and confident obstetric anesthesiologist after completing this fellowship.

Neurosurgical Anesthesiology

Neurosurgical anesthesiology is a 12-month non-accredited fellowship [8]. The program includes extensive exposure to the perioperative care of those undergoing craniotomies, spine surgeries, and interventional radiology cases involving neurovascular procedures. A portion of the fellowship can be dedicated to research time, while the majority of the year will be spent doing complicated neurosurgical cases [1, 8]. Such operations may involve tumors at the base of the skull, procedures involving the sitting position, awake procedures, or cerebral aneurysms. There will also be a focus on the intraoperative monitoring that occurs outside of the anesthetic and the management of patients in these cases with limited medicinal resources.

Fellows can also expect to spend some time in the neurosurgical ICU and learn about the postoperative complications for the given surgical case. Additionally, an anesthesia fellow in the ICU will have a valuable point of view as an integral part of the team.

Organ Transplantation

Organ transplantation fellowships are non-ACGME-accredited programs, usually of 12 months duration, but there are those that offer 2-year programs as well. There are various configurations of this fellowship option. Some programs specifically provide experience in single organ transplantation (e.g., liver only); others provide a broader, but still focused, experience (e.g., abdominal organ transplantation); and finally, some cover the full gamut of the organ transplant continuum (abdominal and chest). Some combine transplantation experience with training for major vascular procedures. Programs may provide transplantation experiences exclusively with adults, pediatric patients, or, occasionally, both.

The balance between clinical and research training is often individualized and based on the fellow's specific plans and goals. Programs that offer 2-year options may include a more complex arrangement with research expectations, adult and pediatric experiences, training in transplantation of multiple organ systems, or a combination of different clinical specialties.

Fellows in an anesthesiology transplantation fellowship should be an integral part of the transplantation team, and, in addition to management of the myriad of pathophysiologic processes associated with various organ failure processes, they should develop solid experience with intraoperative transesophageal echocardiography, clotting status as defined by thromboelastography, and the nuances of transfusion medicine, especially as it relates to reductions in blood product utilization. Trainees will likely gain extensive experience with rapid infusion systems, cell salvaging, veno-veno bypass, and all general forms of anesthesia monitoring. Some fellowships will emphasize perioperative management, including the preoperative evaluation and care of the transplant patient as well as operative and postoperative care.

Regional Anesthesiology

Regional anesthesia is not an accredited fellowship as of 2013. There are a number of fellowship programs that offer 12-month fellowship programs. Although there are no current guidelines for regional fellowship training, recently there has been discussion in formatting a tentative curriculum [4].

This is a subspecialty concentrating on perioperative management of acute pain. Fellows can expect education on peripheral nerve blockade as well as neuraxial analgesia. The clinical program will help fellows learn the indications as well as contraindications and techniques involved in multiple peripheral nerve blocks as well as intermediate blocks like thoracic epidurals and deep cervical blocks. Advanced techniques including continuous blocks as well as some rotations focusing on pain management in patients with chronic pain syndromes can be expected. Multiple didactic sessions will be available as well as journal clubs and research conferences. Additionally, the role as an acute pain consult and collaboration skills will be honed.

Value of Accreditation

Accredited fellowships are those that are overseen by the Accreditation Council for Graduate Medical Education (ACGME). There are 27 Residency Review Committees (RRCs) which vary along all the major specialties as well as for transitional programs. These committees are made up of voluntary physicians that have been appointed by the specific medical specialty organization within that field. In the past, accreditation has been given to each fellowship program with a time-limited range of up to a maximum of 5 years. Programs with shorter accreditation cycles were subject to review more frequently and generally reflected issues that needed to be addressed within the program structure itself. This system is being replaced with the Next Accreditation System (NAS) which will have a substantively different procedure for determining accreditation. This impacts the fellow directly in that the ACGME oversees how the programs are structured and managed, assesses if appropriate education and goals are being met, and regulates various aspects of the work environment, such as the 80 h work week, similar to basic residency programs. Fellowship stipends are comparable to resident stipends but are generally adjusted upward as appropriate for the commensurate PGY level of training. Moonlighting may or may not be allowed, at the discretion of the program director, but work must stay within the 80 h work week limitation. These rules may not be as stringent in fellowships that are non-accredited. Only ACGME-accredited programs receive federal funding for graduate medical education. Fellows must attend an accredited fellowship in order to sit for an ACGME board examination.

Fellowship training must be viewed as an investment in the future. The choice to pursue advanced, subspecialty training has personal, professional, and economic impacts, both positive and negative. This is usually, although not always, the final decision that determines one's professional course throughout one's career and should be made with due consideration and calculations.

References

1. Accreditation Council for Graduate Medical Education. www.ACGME.org
2. American Society of Critical Care Anesthesiologists. www.socca.org/
3. NRMP Fellowship Matches. www.NRMP.org
4. American Society of Regional Anesthesia and Pain Medicine. www.asra.com/
5. Society of Cardiovascular Anesthesiologists. www.scahq.org/
6. Society for Pediatric Anesthesia. www.pedsanesthesia.org
7. Society for Obstetric Anesthesia and Perinatology: SOAP. www.soap.org/
8. Society for Neuroscience in Anesthesiology and Critical Care. www.snacc.org/

Chapter 6
Teaching Clinical Science to Medical Students

Chanannait Paisansathan and Verna L. Baughman

Introduction

Trends in career choice by the US medical school graduates have varied considerably in the past years, with perceived lifestyle and income as major determinants. Medical student interest in anesthesiology underwent a sharp decline in the early 1990s due to the prediction of an oversupply of anesthesiologists. This change led to a severe deficit in the late 1990s, which was followed by an influx of medical students into the specialty during the last decade [1, 2]. Despite the economic downturn in 2008–2010, demand for anesthesiologists is forecasted to continue [2, 3]. The aging population, 2010 healthcare reform legislation, and other substantive healthcare policy changes will likely have a profound effect on the number of operations and interventional procedures performed. Additional medical personnel will be needed—including anesthesiologists—as more Americans obtain health insurance. The uncertainty of healthcare reform, reimbursement, and the competition from non-anesthesiologist practitioners could result in a temporary pause in the US medical students entering anesthesiology during the next several years. However, recent National Resident Matching Program (NRMP) data showed 4.7 % of anesthesiology residency positions were unfilled in 2011, declining to 3.7 % in 2013, in spite of an increase in the number of available positions (from 1,404 in 2011 to 1,653 positions in 2012).

C. Paisansathan, M.D. (✉) • V.L. Baughman, M.D.
Department of Anesthesiology, University of Illinois at Chicago,
1740 W. Taylor Street M/C 515, Chicago, IL 60612, USA
e-mail: oon@uic.edu

Who Do We Teach?

Anesthesiology has grown exponentially in its complexity and practice since the successful demonstration of ether anesthesia in 1846. Additionally, the specialty has been the leading advocate for patient safety and continues to broaden its scope of practice in both perioperative and critical care arenas and especially in pain. Notwithstanding the significant contributions anesthesiology has made to modern medicine, our specialty remains underappreciated. Exposure to anesthesiology during undergraduate medical education is inconsistent and limited, which is a potential factor contributing to the US medical students' lack of interest in pursuing anesthesiology training [4].

Few US medical schools have implemented an anesthesiology clerkship as a requirement, but rather make it available as part of the surgical clerkship or as an elective rotation in the junior/senior year. Frequently an early encounter with the field of anesthesiology results from a student's own personal interest in the specialty. A small number of students have the opportunity to shadow an anesthesiologist during preclinical years or to participate in anesthesia research projects. For these students, inspirational mentors or role models may play an important role in their career choice.

Several common attributes have been identified among medical students who chose to become anesthesiologists: attraction to the clinical application of physiology and pharmacology, pleasure in applying technical skills, desire to focus on one patient at a time, and the wish to control medical care during a critical time in patients' lives [5].

Effective teaching of current medical students requires an understanding of stakeholder characteristics. Different generations adopt distinct motivations and values. Presently, senior faculty belong to the boomer generation (born 1946–1962), mid-level and junior faculty members tend to belong to generation X (born 1963–1981), and current residents, interns, and medical students mostly are in generation Y (born 1982–2000). There is a fundamental difference between the boomer generation and generations X and Y. The older generation considers working hard and loyalty as the cornerstones of their profession, with an expectation of the same from their students. Little dissimilarity exists between generations X and Y. Both of these generations embrace hard work as long as it does not disrupt lifestyle. Time off is highly valued. They support diversity and use technology extensively [6].

Over the years, the number of women admitted to the US medical school has increased to over 50 %. The combination of perceived time flexibility that anesthesiology practice offers and their desire not to postpone childbearing attracts female medical students. A study published in 2012, looking at the factors affecting admission to anesthesiology residency in the United States, pointed toward slight gender bias in favor of women [7]. The common values shared between the female gender and generations X and Y include the desire for mentoring and personal improvement of skills. Thus, understanding these characteristics of our medical students is essential for educators to delineate learning objectives, develop teaching skills, and design appropriate assessment tools for the medical student curriculum.

Implementation of the 80 h work week restriction for residents has created a shortage in resident physician contributions to medical student education, since residents are a major component in medical student teaching. Student education/exposure to anesthesia often depends on pairing with a specific resident for a period of time. Resident work hour restrictions result in disruption of consistent mentorship and can hinder medical student technical skill development. In addition, the implementation of resident duty hour regulations has triggered discussions of similarly restricting medical student work hours. Friedman reported over 80 % of medical schools have existing policies that "define or restrict" student work hours [8]. Thus far, there is no survey evaluating work hours for medical students in anesthesiology or detecting the direct effect of resident work hours on medical student education.

What Do We Teach?

Teaching Domains

The broad spectrum of anesthesiology as the practice of perioperative medicine necessitates a solid foundation of medical knowledge and its application in the clinical setting (analytic and clinical reasoning), perioperative technical skills (self-reflection and improvement), effective interpersonal and communication skills (team work), and professionalism [9–11]. These attributes are consistent with Bloom's taxonomy which divides educational objectives into three similar domains: cognitive (knowledge), psychomotor (skills), and affective (attitudes and value). Thus, teaching anesthesiology clinical science and clinical skills to medical students should include these domains as essential educational rubrics in the medical student curriculum [12, 13] (Table 6.1).

Scope of Practice

The role of anesthesiologist has expanded beyond the operative setting. Preoperative preparation and postoperative management (including acute and chronic pain treatment and critical care) are integrated into anesthesiology and need to be included in medical student education. It is important that medical students

Table 6.1 Teaching domains

Cognitive (knowledge)
Psychomotor (skills)
Analytical and clinical reasoning
Self-reflection and improvement
Teamwork (communication)
Professionalism

understand and experience the range of anesthesia work settings, including operating rooms, labor and delivery suites, ambulatory and procedural clinics, and diagnostic interventional radiology suites. Each setting is accompanied by different environments and workload demands requiring many levels of patient care and interpersonal interactions.

The Anesthesiology Clerkship

Anesthesiology clerkships usually last 2 weeks (regular elective) or 4 weeks (career elective). Both serve the purpose of introducing medical students to anesthesiology. This exposure allows medical students to understand and appreciate the role an anesthesiologist plays in total patient care. It also provides students with real-life experiences of anatomy, physiology, and pharmacology. They participate in the care of patients ranging in age from newborn to geriatric. Because anesthesiology requires a broad-based knowledge of basic science and an extensive understanding of a variety of disease conditions, a majority of the US medical schools require completion of an internal medicine clerkship prior to the anesthesia clerkship. If students come without this background, much of the value of the clerkship is lost.

Clerkship goals and objectives should not only define the introductory knowledge in anesthesiology but also serve as a bridge for successful transition into early residency training. Morgenstern recommends clerkship goals be described by the SMART approach (specific/measurable/achievable/realistic/time bounded) [14]. A common mistake in medical education is trying to teach an overwhelming number of facts and data to the learners in a limited time, which results in short-term memorization instead of learning. Thus, the clerkship curriculum and the organization of clinical teaching have to be focused and realistic [14] (see Table 6.2 for an example of a clerkship educational plan). It must be geared to teach certain predefined goals—and to teach them at a medical student level—not a resident level. Medical students "experience anesthesia" while residents are "invested in anesthesia."

During surgery, anesthesiologists create a condition that permits unawareness, minimizes pain, and maintains physiologic homeostasis while allowing rapid emergence and resumption of normal body function immediately following surgery. Therefore understanding the pharmacokinetic and pharmacodynamic actions of anesthesia drugs decreases medical student anxiety when in the operating room. It is also logical to incorporate into medical student training the concept of pain pathways, their proposed mechanisms of action, and their interactions with multiple drugs. This provides a platform for all physician-directed pain treatments.

Anesthesia apparatus and monitoring systems are everyday tools in anesthesia practice. Understanding the physical principles behind these advance clinical technologies enhances the student's ability to correctly interpret real-time information and make appropriate treatment adjustments to the dynamic changes during surgery. Understanding these functions will benefit medical students regardless of future career selection.

Table 6.2 Example of clerkship educational plan

Week 1
Monday: orientation
Tuesday: lecture—preoperative assessment and airway management
Wednesday: Simulation lab—technical skills (intubation, LMA, IV/arterial lines)
Friday: case presentation by teacher/discussion by students
Week 2
Monday: lecture—pharmacodynamics and pharmacokinetics of anesthesia drugs
Tuesday: lecture—pharmacology of pain medications
Wednesday: Simulation lab—anesthesia induction (IV, inhalational, rapid sequence)
Thursday: journal club (clinical article)
Friday: for 2-week clerkship—oral presentation by each student; written exam
For 4-week clerkship
Week 3
Monday: lecture—fluid and blood administration
Tuesday: lecture—cardiovascular physiology and drug pharmacology
Wednesday: Simulation lab—hypotension (hemorrhage, anaphylaxis)
Friday: computer-based simulation
Week 4
Monday: lecture—ECG review Simulation
Tuesday: journal club (basic science article)
Wednesday: Simulation lab—ACLS
Friday: oral presentation by each student; written exam

How Do We Teach?

There is no consensus regarding the sequencing of anesthesia educational experiences. Do students learn better with an initial formal academic review and then clinical experience, or should the student observe clinical phenomena and then be exposed to formal educational activities? Generally, older anesthesiologists preferred "conventional learning" which emphasized the acquisition of factual knowledge for which immediate clinical application might not be evident. Residents appreciate a more flexible learning format. This refers to the acquisition of a knowledge base needed to explain and manage clinical problems [7, 15].

The classical setting for clinical learning is a medical student's apprenticeship with a resident or attending anesthesiologist in the operating room. Because the operating room environment can be confusing and intimidating, medical students are often baffled about their role and responsibilities, especially in a high-intensity specialty such as anesthesiology, where seconds may alter outcome. Medical students must always introduce themselves to the patients, including the roles they will take in patient care: (1) observation, (2) perform procedures only under direct supervision of the attending anesthesiologists, and (3) discuss perioperative management with the anesthesia team. It is important to orient students to the clinical setting. This is a key step in establishing a positive learning climate.

Teaching occurs in a small group or one-on-one setting. Both allow for active participation between student and teacher. However, in the clinical setting, the learning or assimilation of new knowledge into a preexisting conceptual framework might not fully occur. The burden of work place efficiency, the stress from high standards of patient safety and dynamic changes in the patient's condition may prevent an attending anesthesiologist from completely enlisting medical students as apprentices. This allows only passive learning of clinical management and hinders full engagement from the medical students. Protocol-driven management plans, in an attempt to standardize practice and enhance patient safety, can further dampen analytic and critical thinking. Time constraints from rapid operating room turnover, especially with short cases, may make it difficult to have a meaningful discussion with the medical student and can result in an unintended lack of effective feedback. Occasionally, a poor patient outcome can further dampen a student's ability to self-reflect and to appreciate the learning points from a disturbing clinical event. Thus, the combination of clinical exposure with teaching in a more controlled non-threatened environment, where students do not have the pressure of being rushed into performing or understanding difficult concepts, would benefit students in the development of cognitive skills and maintain self-motivation. The classic example for teaching in this setting is with simulators. Learning with simulation allows students to use both psychomotor and cognitive domains to solve clinical problems. High-fidelity simulations mimic the real patient response, including bad outcomes, which can elicit student psychological responses. Fear and anxiety can present as a high pitch voice, shaking hands, diaphoresis, and palpitation during the session. It is best to develop simulated case scenarios based on real cases and events to add robustness to the learning.

Teaching During the Clinical Setting

The Role of the Clinical Teacher

Besides being an expert in medical knowledge, clinical skills, and clinical reasoning, a good clinical teacher's attributes are enhanced by noncognitive skills. Good teachers develop positive relationships with students and provide a supportive learning environment. Excellent listening and speaking skills allow clinical teachers to encourage active participation, establish rapport, answer questions precisely, and question students in a nonthreatening manner. Being a humane physician who is enthusiastic not only about the practice of medicine but also about the enjoyment of teaching engenders student interest [16]. The intertwined roles of teacher and student are equally relevant for successful learning [17]. Teaching in anesthesiology focuses on engaging students, generating enthusiasm, and promoting a learning environment in a high-intensity setting. This is a herculean task, but it is crucial for our students' education and our specialty's future (Table 6.3).

Table 6.3 Tips to improve clinical teaching

Before/during the case
- Identify learning goals and discuss with student—be specific: technical skills, communication, or knowledge. Focus on one or two goals for each case

At the conclusion of the case
- Ask students to summarize 1–2 learning points from the case
- Encourage students to identify a specific area that can be improved for future performance

Teaching with Questions to Enhance Clinical Reasoning

During clinical case presentations, asking questions is an excellent way to engage medical students and stimulate discussion. It also serves as an evaluation tool for assessing the student's knowledge level and is a good way to monitor student progress. Asking open-ended questions promotes higher-order thinking and encourages refection. Factual questions or lower-order questions do not enhance analytic and critical thinking or problem-solving skill, but they are a useful measure of information recall.

Questions that ask students to summarize, analyze, categorize, compare, contrast, and justify stimulate higher-order thinking. For example, during preoperative assessment, ask a medical student for his/her assessment of an ASA classification for a patient with a history of coronary disease who received two stents several years ago but currently has no chest pain. Then change the situation to a more complex condition but in the same context. For example, ask "what if this patient has some chest discomfort when she plays tennis for 2 h, will that change her ASA classification?" Why/Why not? Using questions is not only a tool for teachers to assess the student's knowledge. It also enables the teacher to identify and clarify areas of confusion, uncertainty, or knowledge deficit. The teacher can help guide the student to select focused, patient-related questions for self-direct learning. This provides the opportunity to include a review of pertinent literature for evidence-based medicine regarding the topic of discussion and encourages the lifelong learning habits.

Teaching Through "Active Observation"

Teaching medical students in the presence of a patient is a delicate process. The teacher has a responsibility to assess the patient's emotional distress related to surgery while also being aware of the learner's ability and skills. A patient's discomfort with the presence of a medical student can translate into a mistrust of the entire anesthesia team, putting the student in a stressful position. It is important to incorporate the patient's approval for their teaching role, usually by obtaining verbal consent. Encourage the patient to give feedback to both you and the medical student [18]. The initial contact between the anesthesiologist and the anxious patient waiting for surgery presents a great opportunity to demonstrate the unique communication skills anesthesiologists possess. It also demonstrates the role of professionalism as a model for medical students.

"Active observation" is an excellent teaching method. Before a patient encounter, the teacher identifies what the student should learn from observing the teacher's interaction with the patient. After identifying the learning objective, tell the student what to pay attention to, in order to create "active observation." For example, a patient with an ASA IVE physical status is about to undergo an exploratory laparotomy for suspected ischemic bowel. The learning objective may be to discuss the do-not-resuscitate (DNR) status with the patient/family and to develop a management plan for the surgery. Direct your medical student to pay attention to the emotional stress level, the acceptance level, and the success of communicating the management plan. After the clinical encounter, discuss what the student observed and learned from watching the anesthesiologist–patient interaction. After listening to their observations, continue the discussion with "how else could we have confirmed that the patient and family understand what perioperative DNR status means and the subsequent ramifications of this status." This promotes higher-order thinking.

Teaching Technical Skills

Teaching procedural skills is crucial for the student's ability to develop both cognitive and psychomotor competencies in order to successfully perform a procedure on a real patient. Anesthesia technical skills should include basic airway skills such as mask ventilation with oral/nasal airway, classical endotracheal intubation using direct laryngoscopy technique, the laryngeal mask airway (LMA), and intravenous catheter placement. The LMA can also be used as an emergency airway device, which is currently taught in basic CPR. Achievement of these skills will be beneficial when the medical student certifies in CPR training and enters internship.

Teaching procedural skills can be broken down into four simple steps (Table 6.4). The first step includes a discussion of the indications and contraindications, the required equipment, and the patient position. Next is a demonstration step. Do the procedure in a slow manner, discussing each step as it is performed. Urge the student to use "direct observation." For example, before an endotracheal intubation,

Table 6.4 Teaching technical skills

1. Discuss indications/contraindications
2. Demonstration of skill
3. Student describes how to do procedure
4. Student performs procedure on a patient with immediate feedback

ask the student to observe the coordination of both hands during application of the laryngoscope blade and motion of the hands while lifting the epiglottis to visualize the vocal cords. When I teach students how to perform an endotracheal intubation, I demonstrate twice. I have them observe the first time. During the second demonstration, the students talk through the steps of the procedure as I perform them. This allows the student to add the motor skill component to the cognitive component. After the demonstration, the student should be able to describe the mechanics of an endotracheal intubation procedure while creating a mental picture of how to perform it. Discussion after demonstration allows the teacher to identify any gaps of understanding which would prevent the student from achieving a successful intubation. Then, students practice intubation using real equipment on an imaginary patient and describe each step while performing it. For the more advanced student, this can include maneuvers required for a difficult intubation. Knowing the steps is as important as hand memory when learning how to perform a new procedure. Similarly, when learning to play tennis, we have to train our muscles how to hold the racket and how to hit backhand or forehand without the ball. The final step is when the student actually performs the procedure. The student should describe each step while they perform them. The teacher can modify the procedure in real time to achieve success. During the final step, the teacher will provide constructive feedback.

Feedback is essential. It provides an opportunity for self-reflection and a plan for self-improvement. Through feedback, students interact and engage with a clinical teacher in order to become more competent. It is not uncommon that the first attempted procedure results in a failure. The student should identify the incorrect step which resulted in failure. The teacher then encourages the student to develop a cognitive plan to solve the problem. Novice students might not be able to effectively do this, so the teacher can use constructive suggestions to guide the thinking process. Constructive feedback should be timely and clear. If done in a timely fashion, students will be able to recall, accept feedback, and make the appropriate modification. Feedback should be on specific performance and not generalized. Table 6.3, summarizes this technique to improve clinical teaching in the clinical setting.

Deliberate practice leads to excellent skills. The relatively short exposure to anesthesiology does not offer students the opportunity to become independent operators, especially for complex skills such as endotracheal intubation.

Teaching Communication Skills and Professionalism

Teaching communication skills is considered an essential part of medical education. Every anesthesiologist works with various personnel, including surgeons, nurses, technicians, pharmacists, administrators, and cleaning staff. Teaching medical students to recognize the complexity of this context and how to communicate effectively is important. A clinical teacher must address this component as part of everyday student learning objective. Direct students to identify an operating room incident that reflects team building behavior and professionalism. Use the feedback session at the end of the day to address this learning objective. After a discussion of what happened and reflecting on how the student feels, a clinical teacher can stimulate thinking about student communication skills by asking questions; for example, Do you agree with what happened and how would you handle it differently? Does it affect patient outcome and in what way? What is the best way to make your point in this situation? Using "passive teaching" in this domain, a clinical teacher serves as a role model for communication skills and professionalism. A student's interaction with a teacher can create a lifelong impression of what he/she aspires to be. As once being students ourselves, it is common we don't remember what teachers taught—but who the teachers were.

Teaching Outside the Clinical Setting

Teaching anesthesia mainly takes place in the operating room. However, teaching outside the clinical setting allows students to gain a greater understanding of various subjects without the stress associated with patient care. For example, teaching procedural skills during a simulation session can be complimentary to teaching the same skills in a clinical setting. Students have the opportunity to practice performing procedures and explore options while doing procedures without fear of causing complications or jeopardizing patient safety.

Traditional Lecture

The traditional 45–60 min lecture remains a mainstay of formal instructional methods. It may be used to provide an introduction to topics that students will encounter during their clerkship. In areas in which students already have general knowledge, a lecture can provide a framework for consolidating that knowledge or restructuring it so that it can be applied in a clinical setting. Lectures are cost-effective and generally are an efficient use of the teacher's time. Lectures can teach a large group of students and cover a lot of content, and many older faculty feel more comfortable with this style of teaching. However, lecturing is a teacher-centered method, and, without careful planning and student "engaging," lecturing can result in teaching without learning.

Certain strategies can be used to modify the formal lecture format to one of active learning and to increase student engagement. A well-organized presentation improves learning and retention. Some organizing principles include the following: *inductive method*—when a real-world example is introduced first, followed by teaching the mechanism underlying the problem or drug treatment; *deductive approach*—starting with the mechanism underlying the concept and then leading to a disease or condition; *time sequence* (*chronological stories*)—people in general enjoy listening to the story, and this approach can promote retention; *pro* and *con*—medical argument can promote engagement and retention; and lastly, *familiar and unfamiliar*—students can relate and help establish the context in which the material fits.

Visual aids are now mostly computerized. Classrooms may have a white board or a computerized white board which can be used in conjunction with a slide (PowerPoint) presentation. The slides should not be overcrowded with content. Graphs, pictures, and videos (either animated or real clinical clips such as an echocardiogram) can enhance student understanding of complicated concepts.

In general, asking questions is a good way to engage student and keep their attention. Lecturer can also use body language, make expressive gestures, move around the room, deliver points from different locations, make eye contact with students, call students by name, vary presentation style, and use humor to keep student attention. An interesting technology to involve students, assess their prior knowledge, and determine whether or not they are learning the material is the use of an Audience Response System (ARS). The lecturer poses a question, and the system electronically collects individual student answers and displays the total response. This describes group knowledge but does not identify specific students, therefore preventing individual embarrassment. This requires a modest financial commitment for the technology. Unfortunately, despite an enthusiastic lecturer, student attention can wean significantly after 15 min.

Team-Based Learning

Team-based learning (TBL) is a peer-teaching method that divides a large group of students into small groups. TBL can be used to teach teamwork and professionalism. Students gain experience working in teams and experience how team-based activity may surpass individual performance. This perspective is important and applies to all aspects of medicine.

After presentation of a problem, each team member is given a specific assignment. Each assignment is important in team learning. The teacher should carefully distribute assignments instead of allowing students to self-assign. Each team should be comprised of 5–7 students and that team should be permanent throughout the course. There are three phases to TBL: student preparation, readiness assurance, and application. During the first phase, students complete their assignments through self-study, reading, and attending educational sessions. The teacher should guide the student though learning objectives, provide a list of suggested readings, and be clear as to the depth of the content. At the beginning of the session, students will complete two assessments (readiness assurance). The first is an individual test (I-RAT) and the second test is a group test (G-RAT). Both tests are the same. Students need to defend their individual answers according to their preparation, and then come up with the group answer/agreement. If there are concerns about the ambiguous questions, students are allowed to prepare a written appeal (feedback). If personal intra-group difficulties occur, it is better to allow the group to sort out its own problem.

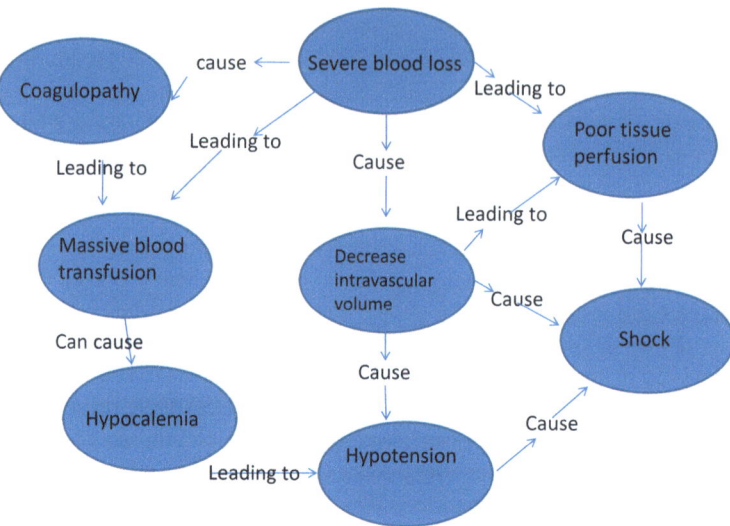

Fig. 6.1 Example of a concept map

However, the teacher needs to closely monitor and should intervene to keep the group on focus. Conflict that needs to be actively managed includes students taking too much or too little time to discuss or students who become disruptive because of poor communication [19]. Finally, the teacher will lead a discussion, offer some immediate clarification (mini-lecture) based on deficiencies found on the test or from feedback. The last phase is application of the knowledge learned during the preparation and readiness assurance phase to solve problems in an exercise known as "Application Exercise," normally a clinical problem. Students must follow the 4 s rule: *significant* to the student, *same* for all students, student required to make a *specific* choice, and to report it *simultaneously*.

Focused Topic Discussion

This method of teaching uses focused topic discussions which can be led either by the teacher or by a student. Teaching in a small group allows face-to-face contact and active participation from learners. The presenter begins with a case description or a clinical problem and then facilitates discussion of the topic. This teaching technique provides a great opportunity for the anesthesia teacher to link basic science to its clinical application. The use of concept maps (Fig. 6.1) in focused topic discussion can graphically reinforce discussion points and explicitly demonstrate thought processes. To create a concept map, students engage in an active process that includes the following steps. First, students identify general concepts and place them at the top of the map. Second, students identify more specific concepts that link to the general concepts. Third, students tie together the general and specific concepts with related words that make sense given the content. Lastly, students actively look for cross-linkages that tie concepts from one side of the map to concepts on the other. Concept mapping has shown to increase knowledge retention in students studying physiology and biochemistry [20] and even in groups with mixed levels of knowledge [21]. In a 2010 literature review, Daley concluded that concept maps are used successfully in medical education because they function in four main ways: by promoting meaningful learning, by providing an additional resource for learning, by enabling teachers to provide feedback to medical students, and by conducting assessment of learning and performance [22]. West, however, favored the use of concept mapping as a learning tool but not as an assessment tool [23]. The strength of focused topic discussions is that they are generally case-based or related to plausible clinical encounters which encourage students to apply knowledge actively. The discussion can promote cooperation and collaboration within the group as it solves a clinical problem.

Problem-Based Learning

This teaching method can be used effectively as a small group activity (ideally four to six members). The session starts with a clinical problem. Students develop hypotheses based on the facts, and then they develop their own learning objectives and plan for solving the clinical problem. This technique is based on a learner-centered approach. With good execution, it is another technique to help students gain both basic science and clinical knowledge through self-learning [24]. Students delegate assignments among team members. Generally, problem-based learning (PBL) continues for more than one session to allow adequate time for students to do research and preparation before returning for a subsequent session. The teacher functions as a facilitator, not to dispense knowledge. The teacher must allow each student to be a teacher and to lead a discussion. Some clinical teachers who are unfamiliar with this method find it uncomfortable. Development of effective PBL cases can be quite challenging and time-consuming. The knowledge acquired from this learning method has not appeared to be superior to other teaching techniques, but it does prepare students for self-learning, which is necessary for lifelong learning skills in physician.

Simulation Teaching

Simulation is the interactive approach of teaching and learning. It offers the opportunity to learn from failure, without endangering patient safety. It also provides positive reinforcement for learned knowledge and skills. Knowledge acquisition occurs through experiencing a reproducible real situation. Simulation tools used in medical education vary from relatively simple tasks such as screen-based computer simulators and low-tech mannequins for practicing simple maneuvers up to realistic patient high-fidelity simulators, which are complex with correct anatomy and physiology. Students engage in experiential learning, using both cognitive and psychomotor skills for knowledge acquisition. Sakawi et al. report increased student comfort levels and success with procedures following stimulation learning prior to patient encounters (in airway management and intravenous access) [25]. Four specific components should be included in simulation sessions: (1) an introduction to the simulation session, (2) the simulation itself, (3) the debriefing, and (4) the evaluation. The introduction is an opportunity for the teacher to set the ground rules and objectives for the session. It is important to keep the environment friendly and supportive, especially during an introduction and debriefing.

Teaching through simulation needs a faculty development program and departmental financial support. High-fidelity simulation provides excellent opportunities to teach clinical reasoning, to help students integrate basic science and clinical sciences [26] in a safe environment, and to expand interprofessional communication among healthcare professionals.

Fun and Games

Learning through games can be an effective and creative way of engaging medical students. It is also a good break from other types of didactic activity. Students can assess their factual knowledge and receive instant feedback. It is important for the teacher to set ground rules at the beginning of the game. These include instructions for playing the game and an expectation of teamwork within the group. Different types of games that can be effectively used are Jeopardy and board games. It is important not to overemphasize the competition among students and corrupt the whole learning experience.

Teaching with Technology Tools

There is an increasing interest in combining the use of technology in teaching. Students learn more from graphics and words than from words alone. Relevant graphics include photographs, animations, and short video clips, which can greatly enhance attention and learning. New information can process to working memory via the separate visual and auditory pathways. Learning is maximized when both pathways are activated. However, redundant information, for example, a teacher reading from slides, can impair rather than enhance learning. Online quizzes can be used as tools to review concepts and to strengthen self-assessment. Video podcast lectures are useful in reinforcing learning and in reviewing [27]. There are several web pages and apps in anesthesiology that can assist both teacher and students as other sources of information. Teachers can use online communities such as blogs, wikis, and interactive discussion boards to communicate with students at different locations. In a virtual equivalent of face-to-face teaching, students can interact to share experiences and information and to learn collaboratively [28].

Medical Missions

Medical student experience during medical missions extends well beyond caring for surgical patients in resource-poor settings. It also involves the training of local healthcare professionals, identification of patient safety concerns, discussion of possible solutions, and implementation of a process that provides for continuing care. This enhances medical student education and appreciation of their role in the global scale of health care.

Evaluation

Evaluation and feedback are essential to the process of learning [14]. Many evaluation tools have been developed to assess medical student achievement. Students learn better if they know they will be tested. Therefore, a carefully thought-out evaluation program is essential for teaching basic science knowledge, clinical application of this knowledge, acquisition of clinical skills, and applying this knowledge to provide safe patient care. It is absolutely necessary that the evaluation process test the predefined goals and objectives. Morgenstern recommends the SMART approach (specific/measurable/achievable/realistic/time bounded) [14].

Multiple evaluation methodologies can be used including written exams, oral exams, case presentations, simulation success, observation of student interaction with a patient, and understanding/achievement of technical skills. The type of evaluation must be described to the students early in the clerkship. Evaluations should be educational, and this mandates interactive feedback with the student. Another important part of evaluation includes the student's opinion of his clerkship. This provides the clerkship director with information necessary to modify and/or reinforce various aspects of the clerkship experience to enhance medical student education.

Summary

Teaching the clinical science of anesthesiology to medical students is challenging. Clinical teachers are faced with generational differences, vast amounts of basic science, and clinical correlations to convey while consistently maintaining high-quality patient care. The nature of anesthesia practice is demanding. It can be stressful for novice learners and for clinical teachers alike. Thus, carefully designed goals/objectives and teaching strategies are imperative. An innovative medical student teaching program and a successful introduction to our specialty are essential to secure the future of our specialty.

References

1. Newton DA, Grayson MS. Trends in career choice by US medical school graduates. JAMA. 2003;290(9):1179–82.
2. Schubert A, Eckhout GV, Ngo AL, Tremper KK, Peterson MD. Status of the anesthesia workforce in 2011: evolution during the last decade and future outlook. Anesth Analg. 2012;115(2):407–27.
3. Levin KJ, Friedman CP, Scott PV. Anesthesiology and the graduating medical student: a national survey. Anesth Analg. 1979;58(3):201–7.
4. Yang H, Wilson-Yang K, Raymer K. Recruitment in anaesthesia: results of two national surveys. Can J Anaesth. 1994;41(7):621–7.
5. Wong A. From the front lines: a qualitative study of anesthesiologists' work and professional values. Can J Anaesth. 2011;58(1):108–17.
6. Shangraw RE, Whitten CW. Managing intergenerational differences in academic anesthesiology. Curr Opin Anaesthesiol. 2007;20(6):558–63.
7. De Oliveira GSJ, Akikwala T, Kendall MC, Fitzgerald PC, Sullivan JT, Zell C, et al. Factors affecting admission to anesthesiology residency in the United States: choosing the future of our specialty. Anesthesiology. 2012;117(2):243–51.
8. Friedman E, Karani R, Fallar R. Regulation of medical student work hours: a national survey of deans. Acad Med. 2011;86(1):30–3.
9. Bould MD, Naik VN, Hamstra SJ. Review article: new directions in medical education related to anesthesiology and perioperative medicine. Can J Anaesth. 2012;59(2):136–50.
10. Michels ME, Evans DE, Blok GA. What is a clinical skill? Searching for order in chaos through a modified Delphi process. Med Teach. 2012;34(8):e573–81.
11. Miller DR. Special theme issue on advances in education in anesthesiology. Can J Anaesth. 2012;59(2):127–31.
12. Teo AR, Harleman E, O'sullivan PS, Maa J. The key role of a transition course in preparing medical students for internship. Acad Med. 2011;86(7):860–5.
13. Walling A, Merando A. The fourth year of medical education: a literature review. Acad Med. 2010;85(11):1698–704.
14. Morgenstern BZ, editor. Guidebook for clerkship directors. 4th ed. North Syracuse, NY: Gegensatz Press; 2012.
15. Filho GR, Schonhorst L. Attitudes of residents and anesthesiologists toward basic sciences. Anesth Analg. 2006;103(1):137–43, table of contents.
16. Sutkin G, Wagner E, Harris I, Schiffer R. What makes a good clinical teacher in medicine? A review of the literature. Acad Med. 2008;83(5):452–66.
17. Karakitsiou DE, Markou A, Kyriakou P, Pieri M, Abuaita M, Bourousis E, et al. The good student is more than a listener—the 12 + 1 roles of the medical student. Med Teach. 2012;34(1):e1–8.
18. Riddle JM. An introduction to medical teaching. In: Jeffries WB, Huggett KN, editors. An introduction to medical teaching. New York: Springer; 2010.
19. Kitchen M. Facilitating small groups: how to encourage student learning. Clin Teach. 2012;9(1):3–8.
20. Surapaneni KM, Tekian A. Concept mapping enhances learning of biochemistry. Med Educ Online. 2013;18:1–4.

21. Richards J, Schwartzstein R, Irish J, Almeida J, Roberts D. Clinical physiology grand rounds. Clin Teach. 2013;10(2):88–93.
22. Daley BJ, Torre DM. Concept maps in medical education: an analytical literature review. Med Educ. 2010;44(5):440–8.
23. West DC, Pomeroy JR, Park JK, Gerstenberger EA, Sandoval J. Critical thinking in graduate medical education: a role for concept mapping assessment? JAMA. 2000;284(9):1105–10.
24. O'Neill PA. The role of basic sciences in a problem-based learning clinical curriculum. Med Educ. 2000;34(8):608–13.
25. Sakawi Y, Vetter TR. Airway management and vascular access simulation during a medical student rotation. Clin Teach. 2011;8(1):48–51.
26. Harris DM, Ryan K, Rabuck C. Using a high-fidelity patient simulator with first-year medical students to facilitate learning of cardiovascular function curves. Adv Physiol Educ. 2012;36(3):213–9.
27. Kannan J, Kurup V. Blended learning in anesthesia education: current state and future model. Curr Opin Anaesthesiol. 2012;25(6):692–8.
28. Chu LF, Erlendson MJ, Sun JS, Clemenson AM, Martin P, Eng RL. Information technology and its role in anaesthesia training and continuing medical education. Best Pract Res Clin Anaesthesiol. 2012;26(1):33–53.

Chapter 7
Mentorship in Anesthesia

Monica S. Vavilala and Elizabeth A.M. Frost

Background

In Greek mythology, Mentor was the son of Alcimus and or Anchialus or Heracles and Asopis. He was a friend of Odysseus who placed him and Odysseus' foster brother Eumaeus in charge of the latter's son Telemachus and of his palace, when Odysseus left for the Trojan Wars (Merriam Webster Dictionary m-w.com).

Because of Mentor's relationship with Telemachus, the personal name *Mentor* has been adopted in English as a term meaning someone who imparts wisdom to and shares knowledge with a less-experienced colleague.

The word "mentor" first appeared in modern usage in a 1699 book entitled *Les Aventures de Télémaque*, by the French writer François Fénelon [1]. In the book the lead character is that of Mentor. This book was very popular during the eighteenth century, and the modern application of the term can be traced to this publication.

Throughout colonial times, it was the custom for aristocratic families to hire a specially trained individual to instruct their sons in politics, Greek and Latin, and the arts. Daughters were also assigned a companion who would instruct them in all aspects of household management and social grace so that as young ladies the former could take their place in society and continue the traditions of their parents. These teachers were also friends to the children and stayed with them, often day and night, until they reached adulthood.

M.S. Vavilala, M.D.
Department of Anesthesiology & Pain Medicine, University of Washington,
1959 NE Pacific Street, BB-1469, Box 356540, Seattle, WA 98195-6540, USA
e-mail: vavilala@u.washington.edu

E.A.M. Frost, M.D. (✉)
Icahn Medical Center at Mount Sinai, 1 Gustav L Levy Place,
KCC 8-46, Box 1010, New York, NY, USA
e-mail: elzfrost@aol.com

While mentorship has been shown to be an integral part of training in anesthesia, and despite its promotion in many departments, there is little published in its support or even in evaluation of its effectiveness [2].

Successful mentorship in academic departments of anesthesiology today can be divided into several component parts: concept, need, identification of individuals who should be mentored, barriers, and opportunities.

Concept

Today, mentorship can be defined as dynamic and developmental partnerships that facilitate the transfer of knowledge, skills, abilities, information, and perspective to foster personal and professional growth. The roles of a mentor are many and outlined in Table 7.1.

A mentor must first of all motivate. From there, he/she can lead by example and inspire, by a role as either coach or mentor. The overall concept is to develop teamwork through vision with an ultimate goal of a win/win situation for all involved.

There are, however, differences between coach and mentor as illustrated in Table 7.2.

Moreover there are several types of mentorship that depend on the circumstance or opportunity as well as many other situations as shown in Table 7.3.

Table 7.1 Several roles for a successful mentor are shown

Teacher
Sponsor
Advisor
Role model
Confidant
Coach

Table 7.2 Several differences in concept are seen between coach and mentor although occasions may call for blurring of the lines

Coach vs. mentor	
Coach	Mentor
• Short term	• Long term
• Performance-driven	• Development-driven
• Task-oriented	• Relationship-oriented
• Design not necessary	• Design always necessary
• Manager is partner	• Manager seldom partner

Table 7.3 Mentorships must afford flexibility to the individual and may also change over time

Mentorship types
• Formal or informal
• Traditional (career) or project-specific
• Rotational (residents)
• Peer (advice)
• Flash (speed)
• Reverse

Establishing the Need

As noted above, despite the obvious need to foster mentorship, little is known about its role in anesthesia and few departments appear to have structured programs [2, 3]. Without a balanced approach to research and investigation and thus progress, anesthesiology risks becoming only a service and purely technical job that could be accomplished by others of lesser training than the many years currently required for the physician anesthesiologist. Schwinn has gone so far as to note that the limited growth in peer-reviewed grant funding and the projected increased clinical demands in anesthesiology now threaten our status as a respected discipline in academic medicine [4]. Without consistent and high-quality mentorship, our growth as academic and healthcare leaders may be restricted [4].

Several studies have, however, looked at mentorship in academic medicine in general [5–8]. As DeCastro et al. noted, career development award programs often require the formal establishment of mentoring relationship, a system that also pertains in anesthesiology [5]. During telephone interviews with 16 faculty members about their experiences with mentoring, Jackson et al. found that 98 % of participants identified lack of mentoring as the first (42 %) or second (56 %) most important factor hindering career progress in academic medicine [7]. While little research has been done on the effects of mentorship on the careers of clinician educators, this group has a lower scholarly productivity rate than the typical research-based educator [6]. One might assume that this discrepancy is related to the need of the clinician to generate income from patient care. However, despite an enormous decrease in grant funding for basic science, researchers still significantly outstrip clinicians in publication rates. The structure of the typical laboratory is geared to a mentorship relationship that could be incorporated in the clinical setting with an association between attendings and residents and fellows but is frequently not seen.

Certainly challenges exist within academic medicine around ensuring clinicians receive appropriate mentorship. Strategies to enhance the mentorship process include the development of formal mentorship initiatives, the creation of workshops organized by funding agencies in partnership with universities, and the development and evaluation of a mentorship training initiative for mentors and mentees [8]. These findings can be applied also to a department of anesthesiology.

A positive role for mentors is in aiding and guiding the publication process. Nevertheless, professional rejection is a frequent experience in any academic medical career. DeCastro et al. conducted in-depth telephone interviews with 100 former recipients of National Institutes of Health mentored career development awards along with 28 of their mentors [9]. The respondents described their experiences with criticism and rejection during their careers, emphasizing the acute need for persistence and resilience in the face of such challenges. The participants described a range of emotional and behavioral responses to their experiences of professional rejection. These responses underscored the important roles that factors such as mentoring and gender have played in shaping the ultimate influence of rejection on specific mentor careers and on the careers of the mentees. While responses to rejection vary, negative responses can lead promising individuals to abandon careers in academic medicine. Resilience, however, can be learned. Given the frequency of rejection in academic medicine, training mentors to foster resilience may be particularly helpful in improving faculty retention in academic medicine.

But while mentoring is central to academic medicine, it is challenged by increased clinical, administrative, research, and other educational demands on medical faculty, not least of which may be instruction in medical schools. Thus, its value and therefore need must be demonstrated [10]. Sambunjak et al. identified all studies evaluating the effect of mentoring on career choices and academic advancement among medical students and physicians [10]. Their search identified 3,640 citations with retrieval of 142 full-text articles for assessment. From these, 42 articles describing 39 studies were selected for review. Less than 50 % of medical students and in some fields less than 20 % of faculty members had a mentor. Women perceived that they had more difficulty finding mentors than their male colleagues. Mentorship was reported to have an important influence on personal development, career guidance, career choice, and research productivity, including publication and grant success although the evidence to support this perception is not strong. Further evidence-based studies with larger numbers are clearly required.

Ethnic minority faculty members are notably underrepresented in academia. However, advancement of these individuals is essential as their research emphasis frequently targets health disparities. Viets et al. describes a culturally centered mentorship program, the Southwest Addictions Research Group (SARG, 2003–2007) at the University of New Mexico (UNM) [11]. The program utilized resources from both UNM Institute of Public Health and its Center on Alcoholism in providing regular research meeting, symposia, pilot projects, and conference support. Positive outcomes were realized by mentee increase in grant submissions, publications, and presentations. Focus-group qualitative data highlighted program and institutional barriers as well as successes that became evident during the program. Based on this evaluation, a Culturally Centered Mentorship Model (CCMM) emerged. Such a program could certainly be adapted and incorporated into anesthesiology training programs where specially selected individuals might collaborate with other institutions in offering expertise and drawing attention to particular avenues through grant support and publications. For example, the New York Academy of Medicine has made major inroads into the care of the poor communities of East Harlem. Anesthesiologists with special interest, training, and guidance could add to these endeavors through efforts in education for preanesthetic preparation and pain management.

It is well recognized that academic physicians, especially early in their careers, lack the skills and knowledge for successful negotiation, regarding it rather as an adversarial process than a necessary and even crucial part of academic success. In a telephone study of 100 former recipients of National Institutes of Health mentored career development awards and 28 of their mentors, Sambuco et al. determined that increasing awareness of alternative negotiation techniques ("principled negotiation") was essential [12]. Shared interests, mutually satisfying options, and fair standards should be emphasized in a mentored setting to encourage the success of medical faculty, especially women.

And yet another need for mentorship was indicated in a recent article. Noting that there is a scourge of academic misconduct, Ochroch and Eckenhoff identified the mentor as someone of primary importance in preventing ethical misconduct [13]. New faculty may find the academic environment overwhelming. While clinical competence is assumed, recognition and promotion with salary increase is closely linked to scholarship. The mentor as an educator is in an excellent position to put the necessary requirements into perspective and help the mentee avoid the many pitfalls of plagiarism. He/she can act as a role model, especially as it relates to research ethics. Also, while junior faculty is often hired for clinical ability, these physicians may have had no training in research or even in seeking answers to clinical rather than basic science questions. Mentors can help these young anesthesiologists develop the required skills and forge academic careers suited to their interests, skills, and abilities.

Who Should Be Mentored?

As Dr. Schwinn noted, successful mentors should enable the best of our mentees to take their rightful place on the stage of scientific discovery [4]. However, given that not all experienced anesthesiologists are suited to mentorship and many residents, fellows, and junior faculty are not interested in further academic pursuits, who should be mentored, and by whom, and for how long? Moreover, as the study by DeCastro showed, many respondents emphasized the improbability of finding a single person who can fulfill the diverse needs of another individual and described the need to cultivate more than one mentor [5]. Participants in the study discussed the use of peer mentors to add benefits such as pooled resources and mutual learning. The conclusion from a nuanced understanding of mentoring from the perspective of a diverse national sample of faculty clinician-researchers was that those who wish to promote faculty careers should focus rather on developing mentoring networks rather than hierarchal mentoring dyads.

The majority of anesthesiologists in training as in the business world are what might be termed as middle-base or B-players. It might be argued that mentoring in a limited market should be reserved for the high achievers. However, certainly in the corporate world, B-players bring depth and stability to companies and improve both overall performance and organizational resilience. These employees will never garner the most revenue or the biggest clients, but they also will be less likely to embarrass the company or quit. In other words they are the backbone of the organization. The long-term performance and survival of any organization depends far more on the contributions of B-players who are able to stabilize the actions of the A-players (high-performing visionaries, whose strengths can lead to reckless behavior). Thus investing in a mentoring program for high performers does not yield as significant a return as might be assumed. Rather, the better investment would be to spend the money on lower performers to help them raise their level of performance [14, 15].

It would appear prudent to offer some degree of mentoring to all trainees, from help with negotiations to project development and grant submissions. Mentoring needs will differ at several stages of anyone's career. Departments of anesthesiology must be flexible and identify faculty who can reliably step in and help at appropriate times.

Are Mentoring Programs Effective: Can This Be Measured?

In probably the first, well-structured assessment of mentorship programs, Farag and colleagues prospectively examined the effectiveness of a mentorship program to promote career advancement in anesthesiology. Based on a 1–5 scale with 5 being very important, physicians were asked to complete a questionnaire on the perceived importance of mentorship programs 2 weeks prior to and 3 and 12 months after establishment of the program [16]. Baseline survey results indicated that 71 % of anesthesiologists at an academic tertiary care facility believed that mentoring was important or very important, although only 46 % felt that it had contributed in their careers. A 2-h workshop then reviewed the commitment to mentorship, provided examples of successful programs, suggested means to identify mentors, and explored how support for academic applications could be achieved. The primary goals set for the mentors were to involve mentees in research projects, encourage enrollment in institutional research courses, provide practice oral board examinations, and create participation in state and national anesthesiology societies and meetings. Several programs were then implemented including manuscript review and assistance, weekly research discussions, encouragement for regular mentor/mentee interactions, opportunities to participate in state and national meetings, and the organization and recognition of mentorship participation in the review process. The original and rather simple questionnaire was given again at 3 and 12 months. Approximately 50 % of participants completed all three questionnaires. Little change in perception of mentorship was found over time. Creating mentee/mentor assignments and implementing a formal program for a period of 1 year did not increase the opinion of the participants regarding a positive benefit of mentorship. Providing regular, allotted time for the mentee/mentor pairs to focus on mentorship activities appeared necessary to give the best opportunity for success according to the general consensus. The authors considered that there were limitations to their study, notably the questions that were posed, the understanding that the study might not apply to anesthesiologists at other facilities not so academically oriented, and the time course of 1 year may be insufficient .Although the approach to mentorship was not proven successful in this study, one might speculate that successful implementation of a mentorship program would provide academic and professional benefits over time. Given that there is enormous variation in content, commitment to, and availability of mentorship opportunities in departments of anesthesiology in the United States, provision of and implementation of a standardized curriculum might be expected to be of considerable value. Certainly several business models have

Research Mentor Evaluation Form

Mentor's Name:
Your name:
Your current position:
Date of evaluation:

Please evaluate the Mentor on the following items, using a 4 point scale of 1 being poor and 4 being outstanding.

		Poor			Outstanding
1.	Meets with me regularly	1☐	2☐	3☐	4☐
2.	Provides adequate time for unhurried discussions	1☐	2☐	3☐	4☐
3.	Reviews my work thoughtfully, carefully and constructively	1☐	2☐	3☐	4☐
4.	Promotes original thinking and analysis	1☐	2☐	3☐	4☐
5.	Offers specific suggestions that I can use	1☐	2☐	3☐	4☐
6.	Assists in developing ideas into viable and successful research plans	1☐	2☐	3☐	4☐
7.	Makes me feel comfortable about raising concerns and asking for help	1☐	2☐	3☐	4☐
8.	Gives me constructive feedback on my written documents	1☐	2☐	3☐	4☐
9.	Gives me constructive feedback on my presentations	1☐	2☐	3☐	4☐
10.	Serves as a good role model of professionalism (excellence, integrity, respect, accountability) in science	1☐	2☐	3☐	4☐
11.	Helps me network with professional colleagues in my area of research	1☐	2☐	3☐	4☐
12.	Overall, provides support for my development as an independent investigator	1☐	2☐	3☐	4☐

Fig. 7.1 The evaluation questionnaire used at the University of Washington identifies both mentor and mentee. It relies on a 4-point score

shown that employees who had a mentor were, on average, better paid, reached their positions faster, and had greater career satisfaction than their non-mentored counterparts [15, 17]. Mentoring has been shown to facilitate socialization of new hires into organization, reduce turnover, minimize career adjustments, enhance transfer of knowledge and values, and help with transition to retirement [18].

Another aspect in evaluation of mentorship programs comes in review of the mentors which is most commonly done by means of a questionnaire completed by the mentees. A question of bias may be raised here in that it is difficult to weed out personality conflicts that might well alter responses and assessments. Also, a mentee may fear that supplying a negative evaluation could result in a backlash and reciprocal poor review from the mentor. Anonymity is restricted or even nonexistent when the mentor/mentee system is on a one-on-one basis. One example of an evaluation form is shown in Fig. 7.1.

Noting that an effective and comprehensive faculty evaluation system provides both formative and summative data for ongoing faculty development, Berk et al. in conjunction with an ad hoc faculty mentoring committee of the nursing department at the Johns Hopkins University developed two tools to evaluate the effectiveness of the mentoring relationship [19]. The mentorship profile questionnaire (Fig. 7.2) describes the characteristics and outcome measures of the mentoring relationship from the perspective of the mentee and the mentorship effectiveness scale (Fig. 7.3) which is a 12-item, 6-point agree-disagree-format Likert-type rating scale. This latter evaluation looks at 12 behavioral characteristics of the mentee [15, 16]. The data thus obtained provides information for annual faculty evaluation, tenure, and promotion decision making. A triad of faculty evaluation data sources—student ratings,

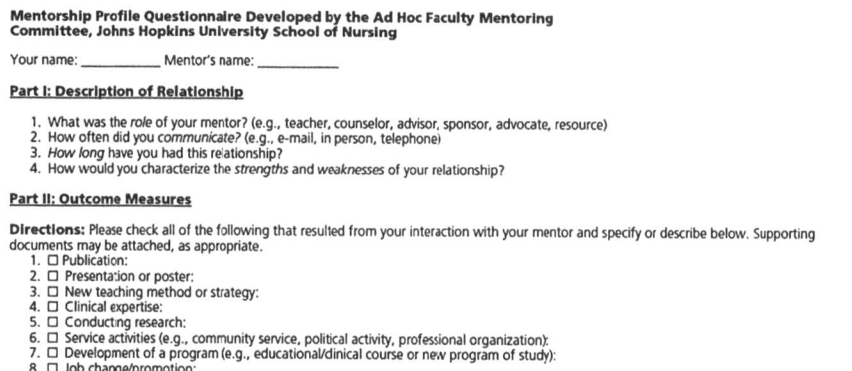

Mentorship Profile Questionnaire Developed by the Ad Hoc Faculty Mentoring Committee, Johns Hopkins University School of Nursing

Your name: _____ Mentor's name: _____

Part I: Description of Relationship

1. What was the *role* of your mentor? (e.g., teacher, counselor, advisor, sponsor, advocate, resource)
2. How often did you *communicate*? (e.g., e-mail, in person, telephone)
3. *How long* have you had this relationship?
4. How would you characterize the *strengths* and *weaknesses* of your relationship?

Part II: Outcome Measures

Directions: Please check all of the following that resulted from your interaction with your mentor and specify or describe below. Supporting documents may be attached, as appropriate.

1. ☐ Publication:
2. ☐ Presentation or poster:
3. ☐ New teaching method or strategy:
4. ☐ Clinical expertise:
5. ☐ Conducting research:
6. ☐ Service activities (e.g., community service, political activity, professional organization):
7. ☐ Development of a program (e.g., educational/clinical course or new program of study):
8. ☐ Job change/promotion:
9. ☐ Grant writing/submission:
10. ☐ Other:

Copyright© 2002 The Johns Hopkins University School of Nursing

Fig. 7.2 A questionnaire designed to evaluate the mentor by the mentee

Mentorship Effectiveness Scale Developed by the Ad Hoc Faculty Mentoring Committee, Johns Hopkins University School of Nursing

Your name: _____

Directions: The purpose of this scale is to evaluate the mentoring characteristics of _____, who has identified you as an individual with whom he/she has had a professional, mentor/mentee relationship. Indicate the extent to which you agree or disagree with each statement listed below. Circle the number that corresponds to your response. Your responses will be kept confidential.

0 = Strongly Disagree (SD)
1 = Disagree (D)
2 = Slightly Disagree (SID)
3 = Slightly Agree (SIA)
4 = Agree (A)
5 = Strongly Agree (SA)
6 = Not Applicable (NA)

	0	1	2	3	4	5	⑥
SAMPLE: My mentor was hilarious.							
	SD	D	SID	SIA	A	SA	NA
1. My mentor was accessible.	0	1	2	3	4	5	6
2. My mentor demonstrated professional integrity.	0	1	2	3	4	5	6
3. My mentor demonstrated content expertise in my area of need.	0	1	2	3	4	5	6
4. My mentor was approachable.	0	1	2	3	4	5	6
5. My mentor was supportive and encouraging.	0	1	2	3	4	5	6
6. My mentor provided constructive and useful critiques of my work.	0	1	2	3	4	5	6
7. My mentor motivated me to improve my work product.	0	1	2	3	4	5	6
8. My mentor was helpful in providing direction and guidance on professional issues (e.g., networking).	0	1	2	3	4	5	6
9. My mentor answered my questions satisfactorily (e.g., timely response, clear, comprehensive).	0	1	2	3	4	5	6
10. My mentor acknowledged my contributions appropriately (e.g., committee contributions, awards).	0	1	2	3	4	5	6
11. My mentor suggested appropriate resources (e.g., experts, electronic contacts, source materials).	0	1	2	3	4	5	6
12. My mentor challenged me to extend my abilities (e.g., risk taking, try a new professional activity, draft a section of an article).	0	1	2	3	4	5	6

Please make additional comments on the back of this sheet.
Copyright© 2002 The Johns Hopkins University School of Nursing

Fig. 7.3 Evaluation of a mentee by the mentor can be made using a scale similar to this one

teaching portfolio, and peer evaluation—are offered [20]. A system of faculty mentorship was implemented, as well as an administrative structure to effectively use data to assist in merit pay and promotion decisions. The authors concluded that using a comprehensive, evidenced-based system to document, analyze, and improve teaching effectiveness is essential to assuring excellence in teaching and learning.

Table 7.4 Difficulties and opposition to the development of mentoring systems come from several sources

- Value/interest
- Incentive
- Recognition
- Good selection of mentors
- Pool of skilled mentors
- Time for mentoring
- Organization and plan

Barriers

Several barriers exist to establishing an effective mentoring program as listed in Table 7.4.

As noted above, no studies to date have validated the effectiveness of mentorship programs, although academicians agree in principle that such programs should be an essential part of training in an academic department. While faculty agree that it would be helpful to have someone to guide in academic and negotiating processes, the time spent to achieve these tasks may be seen as time away from clinical care, requiring that others assume this often arduous load. Moreover, often less or no financial incentive or even recognition is added for those who spend time away from more lucrative pursuits to sponsor an individual who may or may not connect with the visions of the mentor. The mentor may well feel that less than excellent evaluations from the mentee or rejection of a publication or grant proposal may have invalidated his/her efforts and jeopardized a promotion or salary increase. There is little organization or planning that mentorship should and must be part of training in anesthesiology and screening to select appropriate individuals who could be viewed as mentors is generally not in place. As anesthetic administration has become safer, no less in part because of the enormous research that has gone before, coupled with the industry influx of others who have been trained to provide care, many residents on completing training are concerned mainly with joining the most lucrative work force available to repay student loans or support a young or growing family. Such a position, while understandable, is unfortunate and places the specialty in a stationary if not backward position. Only by underscoring the need for guidance towards further research and education can anesthesiology hope to maintain its status in the medical community.

Some Solutions and Opportunities

A start to establishing a mentorship program is outlined in Table 7.5. The curriculum can be based at a grass roots level with anesthesiologists presenting their initial experiences and developing the process from there.

Table 7.5 A mentorship program can involve any members, junior and senior, of a department or departments and should ultimately be a universal part of the curriculum

Starting a mentorship program

• Have one or more persons tell a story of how being a mentor has helped:
   Their department to grow
   They got credit for producing a star performer
   They develop a reputation for caring about people
   How it has enriched their own work experience, career, or life
• Have someone tell a story of how a mentor has helped their own career to succeed
• Let it be known that being a mentor is endorsed by the organization's top leaders
• Give pointers (if possible a workshop, learning session, etc.) on being a mentor
• Do NOT assign people who do not have the time/experience
• Do give small special assignments that will provide a series of small successes
• Discuss opportunities that come with being mentored
• Be generous with praise, but make it specific
• Be clear about your expectations of the mentoring relationship
• Be honest and open when it is not working
• Be able to commit the time and the energy to the relationship

All departments should offer mentorship program correlating the courses with success. Female and underprivileged groups should be specifically addressed. Both clinical and basic areas of research should be identified. Mentors should be recognized and included also from outside departments of anesthesiology to allow for interspecialty collaboration. Mentorship efforts should be recognized and rewarded and workable departmental tools should be developed based at least in part on faculty development reviews that lead to plans. Frequent evaluations at all levels are necessary. Keyser et al. have offered a conceptual framework and self-assessment tool that could assist institutions in advancing their ability to support research [21]. The key domains of research mentorship include establishing criteria for selecting mentors, offering incentives to motivate mentors to serve effectively, identifying factors that facilitate the mentor/mentee relationship, understanding factors that strengthen a mentee's ability to conduct research responsibly, and becoming aware of issues that can contribute to the professional development of both mentor and mentee. Others, acknowledging that current standards of excellence for promotion and tenure are based on outdated models centered on rigid career advancement models, have described an innovative, comprehensive, multipronged initiative based on a promotion/tenure/evaluation system that supports and rewards individual academic career plans. Leadership is also emphasized as is decision making, recognition and rewards for junior faculty, and a deeper administrative and overall team effort [22]. Such an initiative was developed after many meetings with 13 participating departments, indicating the need and benefit for collaboration across specialties.

Other programs have been developed with slightly different aims. A Faculty Mentoring Leadership Program was developed in response to a faculty survey as a peer learning experience for midcareer and senior faculty and scientist mentors to enhance their skills and leadership in mentoring at the Brigham and Women's Hospital [23]. A diverse group of 16 participants met with two co-facilitators in monthly meetings over the course of 9 months. The value of engaging multiple mentors seemed most important. By self-assessment surveys at the start and after 6 months, participants reported substantive gains for mentoring and took steps to build a diverse network of mentoring relationships.

Incorporation of a departmental plan should be given to residents and junior faculty in the form of a letter or agreement by the mentor. Specifically the need for commitment to the program should be laid out. With guidance, the mentee should request a mission and questions with 1-, 3-, or 5-year goals. Mentees should also be apprised of available institutional resources to support their project.

Summary

Although the literature remains limited as to the benefits of mentoring, many anecdotal reports point to its necessity to maintain anesthesiology as a leadership specialty. Value to mentors and mentees are apparent. However, programs should be intentional and integrated and SMART(ER): specific, measurable, achievable, relevant, timely, evaluable, and re-evaluable.

References

1. Roberts A. The origins of the term mentor. Hist Educ Soc Bull. 1999;64:313–29.
2. Flexman AM, Gelb AW. Mentorship in anesthesia. Curr Opin Anaesthesiol. 2011;24:676–81.
3. Flexman AM, Gelb AW. Mentorship in anesthesia: how little we know. Can J Anaesth. 2012;59(3):241–5. doi:10.1007/s12630-011-9657-5.
4. Schwinn DA, Balser JR. Anesthesiology physician scientists in academic medicine: a wake-up call. Anesthesiology. 2006;104:170–8.
5. DeCastro R, Sambuco D, Ubel PA, Stewart A, Jagsi R. Mentor networks in academic medicine: moving beyond a dyadic conception of mentoring for junior faculty researchers. Acad Med. 2013;88(4):488–96.
6. Farrell SE, Digioia NM, Broderick KB, Coates WC. Mentoring for clinician-educators. Acad Emerg Med. 2004;11(12):1346–50.
7. Jackson VA, Palepu A, Szalacha L, Caswell C, Carr PL, Inui T. "Having the right chemistry": a qualitative study of mentoring in academic medicine. Acad Med. 2003;78(3):328–34.
8. Straus SE, Chatur F, Taylor M. Issues in the mentor-mentee relationship in academic medicine: a qualitative study. Acad Med. 2009;84(1):135–9. doi:10.1097/ACM.0b013e31819301ab.
9. DeCastro R, Sambuco D, Ubel PA, Stewart A, Jagsi R. Batting 300 is good: perspectives of faculty researchers and their mentors on rejection, resilience, and persistence in academic medical careers. Acad Med. 2013;88(4):497–504. doi:10.1097/ACM.0b013e318285f3c0.
10. Sambunjak D, Straus SE, Marusić A. Mentoring in academic medicine: a systematic review. JAMA. 2006;296(9):1103–15.
11. Viets VL, Baca C, Verney SP, Venner K, Parker T, Wallerstein N. Reducing health disparities through a culturally centered mentorship program for minority faculty: the Southwest

Addictions Research Group (SARG) experience. Acad Med. 2009;84(8):1118–26. doi:10.1097/ACM.0b013e3181ad1cb1.
12. Sambuco D, Dabrowska A, Decastro R, Stewart A, Ubel PA, Jagsi R. Negotiation in academic medicine: narratives of faculty researchers and their mentors. Acad Med. 2013;88(4):505–11. doi:10.1097/ACM.0b013e318286072b.
13. Ochroch EA, Eckenhoff RG. The role of mentoring in aiding academic integrity. Anesth Analg. 2011;112:732–4.
14. Delong TJ, Vijayaraghavan V. Let's hear it for B-players. Harv Bus Rev. 2003;81(6):96–102, 137.
15. Dickinson K, Jankot T, Gracon H. Sun mentoring: 1996–2009. Sun Microsystems; 2009. Accessed 3 Sept 2009 from http://research.sun.com/techrep/2009/smli_tr-2009-185.pdf.
16. Farag E, Abd-Elsayed AA, Mascha EJ, O'Hara Jr JF. Assessment of an anesthesiology academic department mentorship program. Ochsner J. 2012;12(4):373–8.
17. Roche GR. Much ado about mentors. Harv Bus Rev. 1979;1979:14–28.
18. Kram KE. Mentoring in the workplace. In: Hall DT et al., editors. Career development in organizations. San Francisco: Jossey-Bass; 1986. p. 160–201.
19. Berk RA, Berg J, Mortimer R, Walton-Moss B, Yeo TP. Measuring the effectiveness of faculty mentoring relationships. Acad Med. 2005;80(1):66–71.
20. Appling SE, Naumann PL, Berk RA. Using a faculty evaluation triad to achieve evidence-based teaching. Nurs Health Care Perspect. 2001;22(5):247–51.
21. Keyser DJ, Lakoski JM, Lara-Cinisomo S, Schultz DJ, Williams VL, Zellers DF, Pincus HA. Advancing institutional efforts to support research mentorship: a conceptual framework and self-assessment tool. Acad Med. 2008;83(3):217–25. doi:10.1097/ACM.0b13e318163700a.
22. Pati S, Reum J, Conant E, Tuton LW, Scott P, Abbuhl S, Grisso JA. Tradition meets innovation: transforming academic medical culture at the University of Pennsylvania's Perelman School of Medicine. Acad Med. 2013;88(4):461–4. doi:10.1097/ACM.0b013e3182857f67.
23. Tsen LC, Borus JF, Nadelson CC, Seely EW, Haas A, Fuhlbrigge AL. The development, implementation, and assessment of an innovative faculty mentoring leadership program. Acad Med. 2012;87(12):1757–61. doi:10.1097/ACM.0b013e3182712cff.

Chapter 8
The Process of Board Certification

Ann E. Harman and Cynthia A. Lien

Introduction

Founded in 1938, the mission of the American Board of Anesthesiology (ABA) has been to advance the highest standards of the practice of anesthesiology. Over its 75-year history the ABA has achieved this mission by establishing rigorous standards for what Board-certified anesthesiologists should know and be able to do; developing and operating a national, voluntary assessment system to measure qualified anesthesiologists against these standards; and certifying those anesthesiologists that meet the ABA's standards.

The process of Board certification begins when residents enter their anesthesiology residencies, during which they take the In-Training Examination (ITE) of the ABA, continue through the primary and subspecialty examinations and certification processes required to achieve diplomate status with the ABA, and end with participation in the Maintenance of Certification in Anesthesiology Program (MOCA®), in which all ABA diplomates are expected to participate throughout their careers. In this chapter we will describe the process of Board certification as it unfolds over the course of these three phases of an anesthesiologist's career from residency to retirement.

A.E. Harman, Ph.D.
The American Board of Anesthesiology, Inc., 4208 Six Forks Road,
Suite 1500, Raleigh, NC 27609-5735, USA
e-mail: ann.harman@theABA.org

C.A. Lien, M.D. (✉)
Department of Anesthesiology, New York Presbyterian Hospital, Weill Cornell Medical College, 525 East 68th Street—Room M-312A, New York, NY 10065, USA
e-mail: calien@med.cornell.edu

The Process of Examination Development

The ABA is responsible for the development of several certifying examinations that include the Part 1 Examination, subspecialty certifying examinations, the Maintenance of Certification cognitive examination, subspecialty recertification examinations, and the cognitive examinations for Maintenance of Certification in each subspecialty (MOCA-Subs). While the individuals involved in each examination are different, the overall processes are similar. The process of developing the Part 1, BASIC, and ITEs will be described as an example.

Exam development is overseen by the Joint Council on Anesthesiology Examinations. The Joint Council consists of 14 anesthesiologists, 56 Junior Question Editors, and 32 Senior Question Editors. Junior Question Editors write the majority of new questions each year. These questions are initially reviewed by Senior Editors and revised based on that discussion. All new questions are then reviewed again either at an annual face-to-face meeting or through online meetings of the Senior Editors. Questions in these sessions are reviewed for structure and accuracy and any necessary revisions are incorporated. After being chosen for an examination, each question undergoes another level of review by the members of the Joint Council. During this review, the questions are reviewed for whether they are appropriate for the examination for which they've been chosen, as well as for whether or not they are correct as written. Questions that are found to have errors are returned to the Junior and Senior Editors for revision and replaced with other items that have been similarly reviewed.

The Part 1, BASIC, and ITEs comprise three different types of questions—each with a single best answer. The three types of questions include A—Types, G—Sets, and R—Types. The A-Type questions consist of a single question and a list of 4 or 5 possible answers—only one of which is correct. An example of an A-Type question from the website of the ABA is:

A 60-year-old man is receiving general anesthesia for resection of an abdominal aortic aneurysm. His mixed venous oxygen saturation has increased from 70 to 90 %. Which of the following is the most likely cause for this increase?

A. Decreased cardiac output
B. Intrapulmonary shunting
C. Right to left shunting at the atrial level
D. Wedging of the pulmonary artery catheter*

A G—Set consists of a longer stem that briefly poses a clinical problem. This description is followed by two or three questions that involve management decisions based on the information provided in the original question. An example of a G—Set from the ABA website is:

A young woman with myasthenia gravis was in a motor vehicle crash and requires an ORIF of a femur fracture. Her medications include neostigmine. Her BP is 100/60 mmHg, HR is 120 bpm, RR is 20/min, and T is 36.8 °C.

Weakness associated with myasthenia gravis is caused by which of the following?

A. Decreased release of acetylcholine
B. Increased hydrolysis by butyrylcholinesterase
C. Antibodies to acetylcholine receptors*
D. Proliferation of extrajunctional receptors

The patient's sensitivity to which of the following neuromuscular blocking agents will NOT be increased?

A. Succinylcholine*
B. Cisatracurium
C. Rocuronium
D. Vecuronium

Which of the following *BEST* predicts the patient's need for postoperative ventilation?

A. Preoperative neostigmine dose*
B. Intraoperative use of neuromuscular blocking agents
C. Patient age
D. Duration of surgery

An R—Type question consists of a list of numbered phrases or statements that is then followed by two or three questions or descriptions. The phrase from the list that is most closely associated with that question is selected as the single best answer. An example of an R—Type question set from the ABA website is:

For each patient, select the most likely source of intoxication. Each answer (A–H) may be used once, more than once, or not at all.

A. Salicylate
B. Beta blocker
C. Carbon monoxide
D. Lithium
E. Ethylene glycol
F. Ethanol
G. Organophosphate
H. Tricyclic antidepressant

1. A 28-year-old woman with bursitis presents with diaphoresis, nausea, vomiting, and tinnitus. She is afebrile with a respiratory rate of 36. Blood gas analysis demonstrates metabolic acidosis and respiratory alkalosis. (A)
2. A 60-year-old farmer presents with confusion, weakness, excessive salivation, vomiting, and incontinence of urine and stool. His respiratory rate is 24, he is wheezing, and his pupils are miotic. (G)
3. A 40-year-old man with peripheral neuropathy presents with drowsiness, confusion, nausea, and vomiting. He is tachycardic and has dry mucous membranes. (H)

The In-Training Examination

The ITE is the first ABA examination that residents encounter during residency training. Although the ITE is not a formal part of the ABA's primary certification process, it serves several purposes as it guides residents toward success in the certification process. It allows residents to become familiar with the content and format of the certifying examinations; it allows residents to gauge the adequacy of their growth in knowledge relative to their peers; it allows program directors to monitor and follow the increase in their residents' growth in knowledge over the course of residency training and it provides a means by which resident can study for the certifying examinations. The ITE and Part 1 Examination are built from the same Content Outline and Blueprint. The Content Outline of the Joint Council on Anesthesiology Examinations defines the scope of medical and anesthesia-specific knowledge required to function as a consultant in Anesthesiology and provides the standard of what is expected of a diplomate of the ABA. The Content Outline for primary certification is organized into Basic and Advanced Topics in Anesthesiology. The Basic Topics section contains four subdivisions: Basic Sciences, Clinical Sciences, Organ-Based and Clinical Sciences, and Special Problems or Issues in Anesthesiology. Similarly, the Advanced Topics section contains five subdivisions: Basic Sciences, Clinical Sciences, Organ-Based and Clinical Sciences, Clinical Subspecialties, and Special Problems or Issues in Anesthesiology. Each subdivision contains specific topic areas (Appendix A). The Content Outline is available online at http://www.theaba.org/pdf/Basic-and-Advanced-ContentOutline.pdf and is undergoing frequent revision so that it reflects the current practice of anesthesiology and mirrors certification requirements. Its most recent major revision occurred in 2012.

Historically, the ITE has been a paper and pencil test administered on a single day to all residents throughout the country. As of 2013, it became a web-based examination. It is now offered over a 3-day window at the end of February or beginning of March at each residency program. The ITE is a 4-h examination that contains 225 multiple-choice items and in 2013 the ABA included for the first time items based on moving images such as ultrasound images, patient monitors, and videos from procedures such as laryngoscopy or fiber-optic bronchoscopy. As part of the scoring process, each year's ITE form is equated to a base form of the ITE and examinees' raw scores are converted to the ABA's ITE scale score, which ranges from 0 to 50. This equating process allows programs and residents to meaningfully compare the performance of their residents from year to year. The ABA provides the programs and residents with information about the average performance of all examinees across the country at each level of residency training so that an individual resident's performance can be compared with the performance of all other examinees at the same level of training.

In addition to their scale score, examinees receive a Personal Performance Report, which includes information about their performance on the items in each of the 17 content categories of the Content Outline. The content categories of the report include:

- Anatomy
- Mathematics, Statistics, Computers
- Organ-based Clinical: Cardiovascular
- Organ-based Clinical: Endocrine/Metabolic
- Organ-based Clinical: Hematologic
- Organ-based Clinical: Neurologic/Neuromuscular
- Organ-based Clinical: Renal/Urinary/Electrolytes
- Organ-based Clinical: Respiratory
- Pharmacology
- Physics, Monitoring, & Anesthesia Delivery Devices
- Physiology
- Subspecialties: Critical Care
- Subspecialties: Obstetric Anesthesia
- Subspecialties: Pain
- Subspecialties: Pediatric Anesthesia
- Subspecialties: Regional
- "Generic" Clinical Sciences: Anesthesia Procedures, Methods, Techniques

In each of these categories, the number of questions answered correctly by a resident, as well as the numbers correct in various percentile rankings is provided in the report. Additionally, each item on the ITE is assigned a keyword phrase, which is a concise description of a fact or concept assessed by the item. The Personal Performance Report lists a keyword phrase for each exam item that the examinee answered incorrectly in the content category in which it was included. For example, an item might be aligned to the content category of Anatomy and its associated keyword might be *Celiac plexus blk: Side effects*. This information helps both programs and residents identify specific subject matter within each content area where gaps in knowledge exist and additional study is needed. The full Content Outline for the Part 1, BASIC and ADVANCED Examinations can be downloaded from the website of the ABA.

The Part 1 (Written) Examination

The ABA's examination system for primary certification in anesthesiology currently has two distinct parts: the Part 1 (Written) Examination and the Part 2 (Oral) Examination; each is designed to assess different qualities of a Board-certified anesthesiologist. The Part 1 Examination is primarily a test of cognitive knowledge. The purpose of the Part 1 Examination is to determine whether the candidate has a sufficient fund of general medical knowledge and medical knowledge specifically related to the practice of anesthesiology to be a Board-certified anesthesiologist. The scope of the knowledge tested through the Part 1 Examination is defined in the

ABA's Content Outline, which defines the scope of knowledge that the ABA expects residents to gain during their training in anesthesiology. Residents are eligible to take the Part 1 Examination after successful completion of residency training.

The ABA offers the Part 1 Examination annually in late-July or early-August over 2 consecutive days. It is a computer-based examination that is delivered through the Pearson Virtual University Enterprises (VUE) testing centers across the United States and Canada. The examination consists of 250 multiple-choice questions. The Part 1 Examination is divided into two sections of 125 questions each. Candidates have 2 h and 20 min to complete each section, with an optional 20-min break between sections.

In 2013 the Part 1 Examination included questions based on moving images. The use of these images, screens with vital signs, transesophageal echocardiographic images, and images for ultrasound-guided line placement allows more complete use of the features available through computer-based testing.

The ABA uses an external psychometric firm to score the Part 1 Exam. As part of the scoring process, each year's Part 1 Exam forms are equated to a base form of the Part 1 Exam and candidates' raw scores are converted to the ABA's Part 1 benchmark score scale, which has a mean of 266 and a standard deviation of 50. This equating process ensures that candidates' scores from different exam years are equivalent and can be meaningfully compared.

Once scoring is completed and scores have been verified by ABA staff, candidates receive a Personal Performance Report that includes their total score on the ABA's benchmark scale, as well as their percentile rank. A total scale score of 209 or higher is required to pass the ABA's Part 1 Examination. The percentile rank indicates the percentage of current calibration group candidates who obtained scale scores lower than the candidate's scale score on the current year's Part 1 Examination. For example, if a candidate's percentile rank is 85, it means that 85 % of the current year's calibration group candidates obtained a score that was lower than the candidate's score. Each year's calibration group candidates are all first-time Part 1 examinees that are graduates of American medical schools. The pass rate for those taking the Part 1 Exam for the first time between 2006 and 2012 ranged from 85 to 92 %.

As with the ITE, each item on the Part 1 Exam is aligned to a content category of the Content Outline and has an associated keyword phrase. Like the ITE report, the Part 1 Exam Personal Performance Report also lists a keyword phrase for each exam item that the candidate answered incorrectly. This information is intended to help candidates plan their continuing medical education programs by identifying subject matter with which they were not familiar.

The Part 2 (Oral) Examination

The Part 2 Examination of the ABA is the second examination in the current primary certification process. It complements the Part 1 Examination by measuring attributes of an ABA diplomate that are different than those required for demonstration of a specific knowledge base. Specifically, the Part 2 Examination is designed to test for the presence of qualities and attributes fundamental to performance as a Board-certified anesthesiologist. These qualities and attributes are:

- Judgment—candidates must demonstrate sound judgment and rational thought processes in making and applying decisions; they must demonstrate the ability to assimilate and analyze data in order to arrive at an appropriate treatment plan and to define priorities in the care of a patient.
- Adaptability—candidates must demonstrate the ability to recognize complications and to respond appropriately to them; their adaptability is demonstrated by their ability to respond to changing clinical conditions.
- Clarity of Expression—candidates must demonstrate the ability to effectively organize and present relevant information in a logical and clear manner; they must be able to communicate effectively about issues of specific relevance to anesthesia care and topics of general medicine that are crucial to the care of patients with diverse diseases.
- Application of Knowledge—candidates must demonstrate the ability to effectively apply relevant factual knowledge to management of the specific clinical case scenarios discussed as part of the examination.

To ensure that all Part 2 candidates have the same high quality oral examination experience and the same opportunity to demonstrate that they possess the qualities and attributes required for certification, all Part 2 Examinations are built based on a common Blueprint and the examinations are structured around standardized Guided Questions. The Blueprint defines the content and structure of the examination and ensures that across candidates the examination requires a common breadth as well as depth of information and judgment. Each examination session is structured to ensure that a variety of pre-, intra-, and postoperative topics are discussed and that repetition of topic areas in any examination is minimized.

The standardized Guided Questions provide a brief clinical history of a patient and the examiner uses them to evolve a discussion of the management of that patient. Throughout the discussion candidates are expected to select and defend their plans for patient management. Examiners are looking for clear, consistent, and convincing evidence that the candidate possesses the judgment, adaptability, clarity of expression, and ability to accurately and appropriately apply anesthesia knowledge to the management of a patient's care.

The Part 2 Examination includes two 35-min sessions and two examiners examine candidates during each session. Each examiner independently scores each candidate. Immediately prior to the first exam session the candidate is given 20 min to review and prepare for a discussion of a longer case history. For the second exam session the candidate has 10 min to review and prepare for a discussion of a shorter case history. Each 35-min exam session includes three modules. The modules consist of a set of standardized Guided Questions that focus on different areas in each session of the examination. For the first session the candidate reviews a stem that contains the available preoperative information about a patient. The modules in this session include:

- Intraoperative patient management (10 min)
- Postoperative patient management (15 min)
- Additional topics that are not related to the original case scenario (10 min)

For the second examination session, the candidate reviews a two- or three-sentence stem that briefly outlines the patient's presenting complaints, medical history, medications, and vital signs. The modules in this session include

- The patient's preoperative evaluation (10 min)
- Intraoperative patient management (15 min)
- Additional topics that are not related to the original case scenario (10 min)

For each module the examiners rate candidates based on the evidence presented during the discussions that their judgment, adaptability, clarity of expression, and ability to appropriately apply their knowledge are sufficient to earn the confidence and respect of colleagues and patients. For each topic covered within a module the examiner evaluates the attributes demonstrated by a candidate in responding to questions and describing patient management.

At the conclusion of each module in the session the examiners must determine how often the candidate demonstrated the attributes of an ABA diplomate throughout the discussions of all of the topics in the module. The examiner's Module Rating represents a rating of the candidate's performance and is based on the evidence provided by the candidate while discussing all the topics in the module. The modules are rated using a 4-point Likert scale that includes ratings of Consistently, Often, Occasionally, and Rarely.

Finally, at the conclusion of the entire examination session examiners may also record Deficient Attributes related to the candidate's overall performance during the entire examination session. At the bottom of the Candidate Rating Form (CRF) are listed two Deficient Attributes for each of the four qualities and attributes fundamental to performance as a Board-certified anesthesiologist: application of knowledge, adaptability, judgment, and organization or presentation. Examiners may mark the Deficient Attributes listed as either a "major" or a "minor" deficiency for the candidate. Table 8.1 shows the list of Deficient Attributes as they appear on the CRF.

The ABA uses an external psychometric firm to score the Part 2 Exam. During a typical Part 2 Exam administration week, 950 candidates are examined by approximately 140 examiners. The Part 2 Exam is administered across 32 time periods and candidates are rated on preoperative tasks, postoperative tasks, intraoperative tasks, and additional topics. Candidates receive a total of 12 ratings (two on preoperative, two on postoperative, four on intraoperative, and four on additional topics).

A four-point rating scale is used to rate the candidates on each task: 1 = Consistently demonstrates qualities of an ABA Diplomate, 2 = Often demonstrates qualities of an

Table 8.1 Deficient attributes

Application	Major	Minor
Ineffectively analyzed clinical situations	○	○
Inability to synthesize factual knowledge	○	○
Adaptability		
Inappropriately applied information	○	○
Unable to adapt: changing clinical scenario	○	○
Judgment		
Displayed lack of judgment	○	○
Inappropriate choices of patient management	○	○
Organization/presentation		
Disorganized/unclear presentation	○	○
Provided inadequate information	○	○

ABA Diplomate, 3 = Occasionally demonstrates qualities of an ABA Diplomate, and 4 = Rarely demonstrates qualities of an ABA Diplomate.

The Part 2 Exam is analyzed using the many-facet Rasch model. This measurement model calculates measures of candidate ability, examiner rating severity, and task difficulty. The unit of measure is a logit. The exam is equated to the Part 2 Oral Examination benchmark scale via common examiners and all four tasks. The ABA's benchmark scale and passing standard are regularly reviewed and updated. The current benchmark scale and passing standard were most recently updated in 2012 and the passing standard was determined to be 5.80 logits. This passing standard was based on the Board's expectation that the minimally capable candidate would, on average, often demonstrate qualities of an ABA diplomate across all cases, tasks, and examiners. Logit scores for candidates, examiners, and tasks are converted to the ABA's benchmark score scale and the pass point of 5.80 logits is set to a scaled score of 202 points (the ABA's established standard). In addition to an overall scaled score the candidate's task-level scores are classified as Good, Marginal, or Poor based on the ratings of all the candidate's examiners on each of the four tasks: preoperative assessment, intraoperative management, postoperative care, and additional topics. Once scoring is completed candidates receive a Part 2 Examination Performance Report that includes their overall pass/fail decision, as well as the task rating classification for each of the four tasks. In addition, candidates receive information on the specific attributes that the candidate's examiners indicated were deficient during their examination. The pass rate for those taking the Part 2 Exam for the first time between 2006 and 2012 ranged from 76 to 88 %.

Although achieving passing scores on the ABA's Part 1 and Part 2 Examinations are important steps in the ABA certification process, by themselves they do not guarantee that the candidate will be awarded ABA certification. After successful completion of the Part 1 and Part 2 Examinations the Board reserves the right to make the final determination of whether each candidate meets all of the certification criteria, including the ABA requirements for medical licensure, professional standing, and independent practice. In addition, candidates have a limited amount of time beyond their graduation from residency training to earn Board certification. This time limitation is defined by the ABA's Duration of Candidate Status Policy.

Duration of Candidate Status Policy

On September 21, 2011, the American Board of Medical Specialties (ABMS) adopted a new Board Eligibility policy, which mandates that no more than 7 years can elapse between completion of residency training and becoming Board-certified. The purpose of the new policy is to establish consistency across the 24 ABMS Member Boards regarding the length of time a physician has to complete all requirements for certification after satisfactorily completing training in an ACGME-accredited residency program.

In order to align with the ABMS Board Eligibility policy, the ABA revised its policy on the duration of candidate status. Effective January 1, 2012, physicians that completed residency training prior to January 1, 2012, have until January 1, 2019, to satisfy all requirements for primary certification. Physicians that complete residency training on or after January 1, 2012, must satisfy all requirements for primary certification within 7 years of the last day of the calendar year in which their residency training was completed. So, for example, a physician who graduates from an ACGME-accredited anesthesiology residency training program on June 30, 2014, will have until December 31, 2021, to satisfy all requirements for ABA primary certification. If all requirements for certification are not satisfied within the time prescribed, the physician will no longer be in the ABA's primary certification examination system.

It is important for physicians who are candidates in the ABA's examination system to be aware that the ABA does not recognize "Board Eligible" as a physician status with respect to the examination system. Physicians who are admitted to the examination system are considered candidates in the ABA examination system, not Board Eligible.

Transition to a Staged Examinations System: 2014–2017

Beginning in 2012 the ABA began its transition to a new staged examination system. This new examination system will complement the movement of the Accreditation Council of Graduate Medical Education (ACGME) toward competency-based training and promotion for residency training programs [1]. The first residents involved in this transition include those beginning their internship year in July 2012 and their CA-1 year in July 2013. Rather than taking the ABA's traditional Part 1 Examination, which is administered at the conclusion of residency, these residents and all those beginning residency after them will take two separate computer-based examinations. Each of the two examinations will be administered at different points in their residency training. The first of these examinations, the BASIC Exam, will be offered for the first time in July 2014. Thereafter the BASIC Exam will be offered twice each year in January and July.

Residents who have satisfactorily completed 18 months of training will be eligible to take the BASIC Exam. The BASIC Exam will focus on the basic knowledge required of an anesthesiologist and will include content areas such as pharmacology, physiology, anatomy, anesthesia equipment, and monitoring. The Content Outline that describes the content for the Part 1 and ITEs has been revised into BASIC and ADVANCED sections in order to more accurately describe the material covered in the new examination system. Early and sustained study and learning focused on the basic sciences that support more advanced clinical anesthesia practice are important during residency training. By incorporating the BASIC Exam into its primary certification examination system at the beginning of a resident's CA-2 year, residents will begin to establish sound study habits and acquire more basic knowledge on which to base subspecialty-based training later in their residency experience.

Once residents are in their second year of training, they may take the BASIC Exam every time that it is offered until they pass. After a resident fails the BASIC Exam a second time (or does not take the BASIC Exam on the second opportunity), the residency program is required to assign an unsatisfactory for medical knowledge for that resident for the Clinical Competence Committee (CCC) reporting period in which the exam was administered. In addition, the program will be required to assign the resident an unsatisfactory for medical knowledge for every subsequent CCC reporting period until the resident passes the BASIC Exam. An unsatisfactory for medical knowledge because of failure of the BASIC Exam will require that an overall CCC report of unsatisfactory be submitted. After candidates fail the BASIC Exam for a third time, their training will be extended by 6 months for each CCC reporting period in which they have not passed the BASIC Exam. As a consequence it is not possible for a resident to graduate from residency training without passing the BASIC Exam. However, once residents have achieved a passing score on the BASIC Exam they will have fulfilled the first of four examination requirements toward earning Board certification in anesthesiology.

The second exam in the new staged examination system is the ADVANCED Exam and it will be offered for the first time in July 2016. Thereafter the ADVANCED Exam will be offered twice each year in January and July. Residents who have passed the BASIC Exam and satisfactorily completed 30 months of clinical anesthesia training will be eligible to take the next available ADVANCED Exam. The ADVANCED Examination will focus on clinical aspects of anesthetic practice and will emphasize subspecialty-based practice and advanced clinical issues. ABA candidates who complete residency training on or after June 30, 2016, will remain eligible to take the ADVANCED Exam every time it is offered until they pass it or until the last day of the seventh year after residency training was completed (see Duration of Candidate Status Policy above). Once candidates have achieved a passing score on the ADVANCED Exam they will have fulfilled the second of four examination requirements toward earning Board certification in anesthesiology; they also become immediately eligible to register for the next available APPLIED Exam, which is the third stage in the staged examination system.

The BASIC and ADVANCED Exams will be computer-based exams and each will consist of 200 multiple-choice questions. As with the current ITE and Part 1 Exams, some of the questions will be based on moving images such as ultrasound images, patient monitors, and videos from procedures such as laryngoscopy or fiber-optic bronchoscopy. The BASIC and ADVANCED Exams will be delivered at Pearson VUE testing centers in the United States and Canada. The full Content Outlines for the BASIC and ADVANCED Examinations can be downloaded from the ABA website.

Beginning in 2017 the ABA's current Part 2 (Oral) Examination will be replaced by the APPLIED Examination, which will include both an Objective Structured Clinical Examination (OSCE) component and a standardized oral examination (SOE) component. An assessment center is being developed at the corporate headquarters of the ABA in Raleigh, NC, to accommodate the administration of all APPLIED Examinations. The APPLIED Examination is in the early stages of development. Interested readers should refer to the ABA's website for updated information on the content and structure of the OSCE and SOE components of the new APPLIED Exams.

Candidates will be scheduled to take the OSCE and SOE portions of the APPLIED Exam on the same day, but candidates will receive a separate score for each component. Candidates that fail either component of the APPLIED Exam will remain eligible to retake that component at the next available time it is offered until they pass it or until the last day of the seventh year after their residency training was completed. Candidates that receive a passing score on one of the APPLIED Exam components will have that passing score "banked" and they will retake only the portion of the APPLIED Exam that they did not pass. Once candidates achieve passing scores on both components of the APPLIED Exam they will have fulfilled all of the examination requirements for Board certification in anesthesiology.

Subspecialty Certification

Once certified in the primary specialty of anesthesiology, ABA diplomates may pursue subspecialty certification through the ABA in any of the following five areas of subspecialization:

- Critical Care Medicine
- Pain Medicine
- Hospice and Palliative Medicine
- Sleep Medicine
- Pediatric Anesthesiology

The Critical Care Medicine, Pain Medicine, and Pediatric Anesthesiology examinations are offered through the ABA. Each of these examinations consists of 200 questions and is, like the Part 1 examination, offered as a computer-based examination at a Pearson VUE Center. Candidates for subspecialty certification in any of these three areas have 4 h to complete the examination. Once fellowship training has been completed successfully, the examinations may be taken each time they are offered until the candidate passes the examination. The Critical Care Medicine examination is offered once every other year. The Pain Medicine Examination is offered once each year and the examination for diplomates wishing to become certified in Pediatric Anesthesiology will be offered for the first time in October of 2013. Certifying examinations in Hospice and Palliative Medicine and Sleep Medicine are offered through the American Board of Internal Medicine.

The ABA awards subspecialty certification only to qualified ABA diplomates who do not hold a valid certificate in the same subspecialty from another ABMS Member Board. At the time of subspecialty certification by the ABA, the diplomate must have fulfilled the licensure, subspecialty training, and examination requirements for certification as defined by the ABA. In addition, all candidates for subspecialty certification must be capable of performing independently the entire scope of subspecialty practice without accommodation or with reasonable accommodation and have a professional standing that is satisfactory to the ABA. ABA subspecialty certificates are valid for 10 years after the year the candidate passes the subspecialty examination.

The Maintenance of Certification in Anesthesiology Program

Maintenance of Certification (MOC) is an active process of assessment and continuous professional development that allows participants to demonstrate ongoing competency with advances in the field of medicine throughout their entire careers. The MOC concept originated with the ABMS in 1999. As a member board of the ABMS, the ABA has been charged with implementing MOC activities that will assure the public that its diplomates demonstrate commitment to quality clinical outcomes and patient safety.

Board certification in Anesthesiology is simply the first step in a continuous process of professional development. Diplomates of the ABA must be reflective practitioners who are committed to thinking systematically about their practices and learning from their experiences. Therefore, Maintenance of Certification in Anesthesiology (MOCA®) has been designed to provide ABA diplomates with the opportunity to continuously improve both their knowledge and skills in the six general areas of competency: Medical Knowledge; Patient Care; Practice-Based Learning and Improvement; Professionalism; Interpersonal and Communication Skills; and Systems-Based Practice.

Requirements for each MOCA cycle must be completed during a 10-year period. All ABA diplomates certified after 1999 hold a time-limited certificate and are enrolled in MOCA after initial board certification. Participation in MOCA by non-time-limited diplomates, those certified before 2000, is voluntary and encouraged.

Each MOCA cycle includes activities or requirements in each of the following four parts:

- Part I: Maintaining an acceptable professional standing
- Part II: Obtaining 250 CME credits as part of lifelong learning and self-assessment
- Part III: Passing a cognitive examination
- Part IV: Participating in practice performance assessment and improvement activities

The cognitive examination in MOCA is designed to test general information that should be part of every anesthesiologist's knowledge base, regardless of their area of specialization. As with other ABA examinations, the MOCA exam is computer-based and offered at Pearson VUE testing centers. Diplomates can take the exam as early as the seventh year of their MOCA cycle and they can take it twice each year until they pass it. The exam is offered in July and December of each year.

As with other computer-based examinations taken for ABA certification, the MOCA cognitive consists of a series of multiple-choice, single best answer questions. Candidates have 4 h to answer the 200 questions that comprise this examination. Scoring of the examination is done by an outside testing service. The scores are validated and returned to those who took the examination within 4 weeks of sitting for the exam. As with other ABA examinations, the MOCA exam is a criterion-based examination—which means that if everyone meets the passing standard, everyone passes. In addition to their score, all candidates receive a key word report listing all of the topics addressed incorrectly by the candidate. This year (2013), the ABA will also provide a "Top Twenty Topic" list that will include the 20 topics most frequently addressed incorrectly by candidates. This feedback can be used to guide future study while fulfilling ongoing MOCA requirements or help with preparation for the next examination.

The ABA has developed the MOCA program with a goal that each activity be relevant to a physician's practice, have high impact on the quality and safety of patient care, be patient-centered, and enhance the public's trust in healthcare. The ABA continues to build evidence surrounding the value of MOCA, while keeping in mind that there are three groups that should benefit from the program: the public, health systems, and physicians.

The Maintenance of Certification in Anesthesiology for Subspecialties Program

The transition from subspecialty recertification examinations to the Maintenance of Certification in Anesthesiology for Subspecialties Program (MOCA-SUBS) began on January 1, 2010. Subspecialty recertification examinations are designed to test for the presence of knowledge considered essential for the ABA diplomate to function as a practitioner of the subspecialty at a point in time, while MOCA-SUBS emphasizes a program of continual professional development and practice improvement. The last subspecialty recertification examinations will be administered in 2016, and the first MOCA-SUBS examinations will be administered in 2017.

Diplomates who choose to maintain both their primary certification and a subspecialty certification will benefit from overlapping program requirements as long as all of the activities are completed during each of the 10-year MOCA cycles.

The MOCA-SUBS program requirements mirror those of the MOCA program requirements, with the following exceptions:

1. Some of the required Part 2 Life Long Learning and Self Assessment, Continuing Medical Education (LLSA<CME) activities must be related to the subspecialty certification being maintained.
2. A separate Part 3 Cognitive Examination will need to be completed for each certificate being maintained.
3. The ABA will verify diplomates' clinical activity in the subspecialty.

Test Security

The integrity of the Board's examination system and the validity of its certification decisions are of paramount importance to the Board. For this reason the Board and its examination administration staff follow careful procedures to verify the identity of examinees and ensure that they do not have access to unauthorized materials or information during the examination process. For the Part 1 Examinations, which are delivered through the Pearson VUE test center network, examinees must present a government-issued photo ID, as well as have their photograph taken and provide biometric data, such as their fingerprints or a palm-vein scan before they will be admitted to the examination. For the Part 2 Examinations, which are delivered by ABA staff, examinees also must present a government-issued photo ID.

In addition, the Board maintains a strict Irregular Behavior Policy that forbids any conduct that may jeopardize the integrity or validity of any ABA examination process or result, including but not limited to cheating, misappropriating, copying, or reproducing any element of an examination for personal use or the use of a third-party without the explicit and specific written consent of the ABA. Information about behavior that the Board considers a violation of the integrity of its examination and certification process is sent to all candidates scheduled for examination. Statistical analyses may be conducted to verify observations and reports of suspected irregularities in the conduct of an examination. The examination of any examinee whose conduct is found to have violated or attempted to violate the integrity of the ABA's examination and certification process is invalidated and no results are reported. In addition, the examinee will be subject to punitive action as determined by the Board.

Conclusion

ABA certification is a professional distinction that signifies that an anesthesiologist has demonstrated—through a series of rigorous examinations—that he or she possesses the knowledge and skills needed to provide a high level of anesthesia care. The Board's current assessment system, from the ITEs to the MOCA program, has been designed to ensure that the highest standards of the practice of anesthesiology are maintained throughout the career continuum of an ABA diplomate. In the coming years the ABA will continue to advance its assessment system by introducing a BASIC Examination at the mid-point of residency training in order to encourage early and sustained study by residents of the basic sciences that are the foundation on which the more advanced concepts in clinical anesthesia are built. The ABA also will augment its current oral examination processes by incorporating an OSCE component; this will allow the Board to assess additional qualities, skills, and abilities of those seeking to become diplomates of the ABA.

Reference

1. Nasca TJ, Philbert I, Brigham T, Flynn TC. The next GME accreditation system—rationale and benefits. New Engl J Med. 2012;366(11):1051–6.

Appendix A: BASIC/ADVANCED Content Outline

I. Basic Topics in Anesthesiology

  A. BASIC SCIENCES

    I.A.1 Anatomy
    I.A.2 Physics, Monitoring, and Anesthesia Delivery Devices
    I.A.3 Mathematics
    I.A.4 Pharmacology

  B. CLINICAL SCIENCES: Anesthesia Procedures, Methods, and Techniques

    I.B.1 Evaluation of the Patient and Preoperative Preparation
    I.B.2 Regional Anesthesia
    I.B.3 General Anesthesia
    I.B.4 Monitored Anesthesia Care and Sedation: ASA Guidelines for Sedation, Sedation Guidelines for Non-Anesthesiologists
    I.B.5 Intravenous Fluid Therapy During Anesthesia: Water, Electrolyte, Glucose Requirements and Disposition, Crystalloid vs. Colloid
    I.B.6 Complications (Etiology, Prevention, Treatment)
    I.B.7 Postoperative Period

  C. ORGAN-BASED BASIC AND CLINICAL SCIENCES

    I.C.1 Central and Peripheral Nervous Systems
    I.C.2 Respiratory System
    I.C.3 Cardiovascular System
    I.C.4 Gastrointestinal/Hepatic Systems
    I.C.5 Renal and Urinary Systems/Electrolyte Balance

I.C.6 Hematologic System
I.C.7 Endocrine and Metabolic Systems
I.C.8 Neuromuscular Diseases and Disorders

D. SPECIAL PROBLEMS OR ISSUES IN ANESTHESIOLOGY

I.D.1 Physician Impairment or Disability: Substance Abuse, Fatigue, Aging, Visual and Auditory Impairment, American Disabilities Act
I.D.2 Ethics, Practice Management, and Medicolegal Issues

II. Advanced Topics in Anesthesiology

A. BASIC SCIENCES

II.A.1 Physics, Monitoring, and Anesthesia Delivery Devices
II.A.2 Pharmacology

B. CLINICAL SCIENCES: Anesthesia Procedures, Methods, And Techniques

II.B.1 Regional Anesthesia
II.B.2 Special Techniques

C. Organ-Based Basic and Clinical Sciences

II.C.1 Central and Peripheral Nervous Systems
II.C.2 Respiratory System
II.C.3 Cardiovascular System
II.C.4 Gastrointestinal/Hepatic Systems
II.C.5 Renal and Urinary Systems/Electrolyte Balance
II.C.6 Hematologic System
II.C.7 Endocrine and Metabolic Systems
II.C.8 Neuromuscular Diseases and Disorders: Clinical Science

D. Clinical Subspecialties

II.D.1 Painful Disease States
II.D.2 Pediatric Anesthesia
II.D.3 Obstetric Anesthesia
II.D.4 Otorhinolaryngology (ENT) Anesthesia: Airway Endoscopy; Microlaryngeal Surgery; Laser Surgery, Hazards, Complications (Airway Fires, etc.)
II.D.5 Anesthesia For Plastic Surgery, Liposuction
II.D.6 Anesthesia For Laparoscopic Surgery; Cholecystectomy; Gynecologic Surgery; Gastric Stapling; Hiatus Hernia Repair; Anesthetic Management; Complications
II.D.7 Ophthalmologic Anesthesia, Retrobulbar And Peribulbar Blocks; Open Eye Injuries
II.D.8 Orthopedic Anesthesia; Tourniquet Management, Complications, Regional vs. General Anesthesia
II.D.9 Trauma, Burn Management, Mass Casualty, Biological Warfare

II.D.10 Anesthesia For Ambulatory Surgery
 II.D.11 Geriatric Anesthesia/Aging
 II.D.12 Critical Care

E. Special Problems or Issues in Anesthesiology

 II.E.1 Electroconvulsive Therapy
 II.E.2 Organ Donors: Pathophysiology and Clinical Management
 II.E.3 Radiologic Procedures; CT Scan; MRI-Anesthetic Implications/ Management, Anesthesia in Locations Outside the Operating Rooms

Chapter 9
Maintenance of Certification in Anesthesiology Program

Natalie F. Holt

Background

Concern with the idea of indefinite certification began as early as the 1940s, when it became clear that the rapid advance of medical knowledge made the concept of lifetime certification unrealistic. However, the first time-limited board certifications were not adopted until 1970 by the American Board of Family Practice (now the American Board of Family Medicine). Pediatric surgery became the first surgical specialty to institute 10-year, time-limited certificates in 1973, and by 1976, all American Board of Surgery certificates became time-limited [1].

In 1989, the ABA acknowledged the benefit of establishing a formalized process whereby diplomates could demonstrate continued proficiency in their field. It established the continued demonstration of qualifications (CDQ) program for this purpose [2]. Initially, participation in this predecessor to MOCA was voluntary. In 1995, the ABA approved a proposal to begin issuing time-limited certifications as of January 1, 2000. With this decision, diplomates wishing to maintain certification beyond 10 years would be required to participate in the ABA's CDQ program, which was subsequently renamed recertification. This program included a voluntary recertification examination, the last of which was administered in 2009, when the official transition from recertification to MOCA was completed [2].

In 2000, the 24 Boards compromising the American Board of Medical Specialties (ABMS)—of which the ABA is one—agreed upon a relatively radical restructuring of the recertification process, designed to emphasis not only cognitive proficiency but

---

N.F. Holt, M.D., M.P.H. (✉)
Department of Anesthesiology, Yale University School of Medicine,
New Haven, CT 06520, USA

Department of Anesthesiology, VA Connecticut Healthcare System,
West Haven Campus, West Haven, CT 06516, USA
e-mail: Natalie.holt@post.harvard.edu

also the concept of lifelong learning, self-assessment, and performance improvement. From this discussion, came the four-part MOCA program that exists today. The complete MOCA program became available to diplomates in 2004 [2].

Components of MOCA

MOCA consists of four components, each of which must be satisfactorily completed within the 10-year MOCA cycle in order to ensure maintenance of certification: (1) Part I: Professional standing assessment; (2) Part II: Lifelong Learning and Self-Assessment; (3) Part III: Cognitive Expertise Assessment; and (4) Part IV: Practice Performance Assessment and Improvement.

Part I: Professional Standing Assessment

All diplomates must hold an active, unrestricted medical license in at least one jurisdiction of the United States or Canada. Licensure restrictions are administered by the Medical Board of each state and vary somewhat by region. Examples of actions which typically lead to licensure restrictions include failure to practice within the scope of a licensee's education and training, willful neglect of a patient's health or safety, felony or criminal conviction, sexual misconduct, and presigning of blank prescription forms. If a restriction is placed on a diplomate's medical license, it must be reported to the ABA within 60 days [2].

Part II: Lifelong Learning and Self-Assessment

ABA diplomates are expected to engage in continuing medical education (CME) opportunities throughout the duration of the MOCA cycle, which the ABA calls Lifelong Learning and Self-Assessment (LLSA). The exact number of CME credits required varies based on year in which initial certification was earned (Table 9.1). In 2013, the ABA reduced the number of required CME credits for diplomates certified on or after January 1, 2004 from 350 to 250 to be more consistent with the

Table 9.1 Continuing medical education requirements by year certified

Year certified	Total CME credits	Category 1 CME credits	Minimum to apply for cognitive exam
2001	245	175	140
2002	280	200	160
2003	315	225	180
≥2004	350	250	200

Table 9.2 Practice performance assessment and improvement requirements by year in MOCA cycle

Year certified[a]	1 2 3 4 5	6 7 8 9 10
2000–2003	Attestation	Attestation
2004–2007[b]	Attestation	Case evaluation or simulation
2008 or later	Case evaluation or simulation[c]	Case evaluation or simulation[c]
		Attestation

[a]Diplomates certified between January 1, 2001 and December 31, 2007 have the option of completing a simulation course instead of providing attestation and references
[b]Diplomates certified between January 1, 2004 and December 31, 2007 who choose to complete a simulation course in lieu of an attestation must complete a case evaluation between years 6 and 10
[c]Diplomates must complete both a case evaluation and simulation course during the 10-year MOCA cycle; one activity must be completed during years 1–5 and the other between years 6 and 10

ABMS average of 25 CME credits per calendar year. Therefore, diplomates certified on or after January 1, 2004, must now complete at least 250 CME credits over the 10-year MOCA cycle, all of which must be Category 1 American Council for Continuing Medical Education (ACCME)-accredited activities. Examples of such activities include attendance at meetings sponsored by medical societies such as the American Society of Anesthesiologists (ASA) and completion of educational programs offered in peer-reviewed medical journals [2].

The intent of the LLSA program is to encourage lifelong learning; therefore, in 2006, the ABA established a cap on the number of CME credits it would award per calendar year to encourage diplomates to earn CME credits throughout the MOCA cycle [2]. Until 2012, this cap was 70 credits per calendar year. Effective in 2013, the ceiling was lowered to 60 credits per calendar year [2]. Furthermore, diplomates must participate in CME activities in at least 5 of the 10 years of each MOCA cycle [2]. Many hospitals and some states require documentation of annual or biannual CME activity, which is consistent with the ABA's goal to have diplomates regularly participating in CME programs.

The ABA itself does not offer CME activities; however, all healthcare organizations interested in providing CME programs suitable for MOCA must be approved by the ABA [2]. In addition, the ABA has become more proscriptive in its CME requirements. For example, diplomates who entered the MOCA program between January 1, 2008 and December 31, 2009 are required to complete 60 credits of the ASA's Self-Education and Evaluation (SEE) program and/or the ASA Continuing Education (ACE) program or another ABA-approved self-assessment CME program at least once during their MOCA cycle (Table 9.2) [2]. Diplomates certified on or after January 1, 2010 and those carrying non-time-limited certificates who voluntarily enter the MOCA program are required to complete 90 credits of the ASA's SEE or ACE program or other ABA-approved CME program at least once during their MOCA cycle [2]. In addition, all MOCA participants who entered the program after January 1, 2008 must fulfill at least 20 credits of Patient Safety CME offered through the ASA or the ABMS [2].

Diplomates who complete a 12-month ACGME-accredited subspecialty fellowship or a 12-month anesthesiology subspecialty fellowship in an ACGME-accredited anesthesiology program are entitled to 50 Category 1 CME credits so long as the fellowship is completed in the year of or after primary certification in Anesthesiology is awarded [2]. The ABA does not grant CME credit for fellowships or subspecialty certifications finished prior to primary certification in Anesthesiology.

It is the responsibility of diplomates to report CME activities to the ABA via the ABA portal, which is accessible at the ABA website (www.theABA.org). Furthermore, a minimum number of LLSA credits must be submitted to the ABA by the delegate at least 5 months prior to the examination date for recertification [2].

Part III: Cognitive Examination

Between years 7 and 10 of the MOCA cycle, all diplomates are required to demonstrate core knowledge in anesthesiology by passing an ABA examination for recertification. The examination is a 4-h computer-based test consisting of 200 multiple-choice questions with one best answer [2]. One hundred and fifty of the questions (75 %) are in topics in general anesthesia; the remaining 50 questions (25 %) are divided among pediatric anesthesia, cardiothoracic anesthesia, neuroanesthesia, critical care medicine, obstetrical/gynecologic anesthesia, and pain medicine [2]. Until 2010, the examinee was allowed to answer only 150 of the 200 questions, and leave unanswered 50 questions of the examinee's choice; but currently, all 200 questions must be answered [3]. There is no predetermined passing score on the MOCA Cognitive Exam. However, the ABA reports that since the first MOCA exam was administered in 2005, the pass rate has been greater than 90 % [4].

Prior to taking the examination, diplomates must demonstrate the following three prerequisites: (1) satisfactory professional standing (a.k.a. active, unrestricted license to practice medicine in the United States or Canada); (2) successful completion of half their required CME credits; (3) and one satisfactory Practice Performance Assessment and Improvement Activity (see below) [2].

The MOCA Cognitive Examination is administered twice a year in the winter and summer, and there is no limit to the number of times a diplomate may take the exam. Furthermore, there is no penalty for taking the MOCA Cognitive Examination in years 7–10; in other words, the clock will not restart until after year 10 of the MOCA cycle [2].

Part IV: Practice Performance Assessment and Improvement

The Practice Performance Assessment and Improvement (PPAI) requirement consists of three parts: (1) simulation course; (2) case evaluation; and (3) attestation. Requirements for completion of these activities vary based on year certified (Table 9.3) [2]. Diplomates certified in year 2008 or later are required to complete

Table 9.3 Practice performance assessment and improvement requirements by year in MOCA cycle

Year certified or recertified	1	2	3	4	5	6	7	8	9	10
2003			Attestation						Attestation[b]	
2004–2007[a]			Attestation[b]						Case evaluation or simulation	
2008–2009			Case evaluation or simulation[c]						Case evaluation or simulation[c] Attestation	
2010–2014			Case evaluation or simulation[c]						Case evaluation or simulation[c] Attestation	

[a] Diplomates certified between January 1, 2004 and December 31, 2007 who choose to complete a simulation course in lieu of an attestation must complete a case evaluation between years 6 and 10
[b] Completion of a simulation course is an option instead of providing attestation
[c] Diplomates must complete both a case evaluation and simulation course during the 10-year MOCA cycle; one activity must be completed during years 1–5 and the other between years 6 and 10

an ASA-endorsed simulation education course during the 10-year MOCA cycle. Participation in simulation education is optional for diplomates certified in years 2003–2007. The purpose of simulation training is to provide a context in which to improve skills in areas such as teamwork and communication, crisis management, and clinical emergencies such as the difficult airway, anaphylaxis, and cardiac arrest. Currently, there are 35 ABA-endorsed simulation centers offering courses that meet the MOCA Part IV requirement (see http://www.asahq.org/For-Members/Education-and-Events/Simulation-Education/Endorsed-Simulation-Centers.aspx).

Diplomates certified in years 2004 or later are also required to complete a case evaluation [2]. This is a four-step process intended to allow diplomates to analyze their practice then develop and implement a practice improvement program. This process may be conducted individually or as a group effort, for example among several diplomates who work at the same facility. The improvement initiative is expected to be evidence based and to take one of four forms: a (1) clinical pathway; (2) clinical reminder; (3) personal reminder; or (4) change in system or practice. For example, an anesthesiologist who perceives that patients on beta blockers neglect to take their prescribed dose on the morning of surgery, despite being told to do so in the Preanesthesia Clinic, thinks that a phone call reminding patients to do so would improve compliance. Before any intervention, the anesthesiologist collects data on how many patients on beta blockers actually take their medication on the day of surgery over a 2-week period. Next, a system is implemented in which, while nurses are calling patients to tell them when to arrive for surgery, they also review which medications patients should take that morning. Data is collected over another 2-week period after the intervention. The results demonstrate a 20 % increase in beta blocker use on the morning of surgery in patients on chronic beta blockers, suggesting the intervention helped improve medication compliance. As a result of its success, the change in practice becomes a permanent practice change. Additional examples of case evaluations are available on the ABA website (www.theABA.org).

At least once in each MOCA cycle, the ABA solicits three references submitted by the diplomate and intended to attest to the diplomate's clinical work and participation in practice improvement activities [2]. The diplomate submits the names of the references to the ABA via the ABA portal. The attestation process is due in year 9 of the MOCA cycle.

Voluntary MOCA for Non-Time-Limited Certificate Holders

Diplomates who hold non-time-limited certificates and voluntarily participate in MOCA have the option to complete the program on an expedited basis [2]. The diplomate is asked to report CME from the 10 years prior to MOCA enrollment, and MOCA requirements are adjusted based on the number of years elected to complete the program (minimum of 2 years). If the MOCA program is completed in 5 years or less, only two Part IV activities are required: the attestation and either a case evaluation or simulation course.

It should be noted that although there is no ABA obligation for diplomates with non-time-limited certificates to participate in MOCA, some hospitals require MOCA participation as a condition for granting hospital privileges. In addition, some liability insurers offer a discount to physicians who participate in MOCA components, such as a simulation course [5, 6]. In addition, effective in 2013, participation in MOCA can qualify ABA diplomates for an incentive payment from the Centers for Medicare and Medicaid Services.

MOCA for Subspecialties

The ABA offers subspecialty certification in five disciplines: (1) critical care medicine; (2) pain medicine; (3) hospice and palliative medicine; (4) sleep medicine; and (5) pediatric anesthesiology. Like primary certification in anesthesiology, all subspecialty certifications are now issued on a 10-year time-limited basis. Until 2010, the recertification process involved only a cognitive examination. In January 1, 2010, the ABA began transitioning from subspecialty recertification to the Maintenance of Certification in Anesthesiology for Subspecialties (MOCA-SUBS) program [2]. The last subspecialty recertification examinations will be given in 2016 and the first MOCA-SUBS Examinations will be administered in 2017.

Many of the MOCA and MOCA-SUBS program requirements overlap and may therefore be shared, facilitating the maintenance of both certifications. These requirements include: Part I: Professional standing; Part II: Lifelong Learning and Self-Assessment; and Part IV: Practice Performance Assessment and Improvement [2]. Diplomates who hold one subspecialty certification are required to complete a case evaluation in a subspeciality-related discipline. In addition, a portion of the diplomate's CME must be related to the subspecialty. Separate Part III Cognitive Examinations are required for each certificate being maintained [2].

Diplomates holding time-limited primary and subspecialty certifications are encouraged but not required to maintain both certifications.

Reciprocity for Diplomates with Certifications in Other Specialties

Diplomates who are certified in another specialty recognized by the ABMS are allowed to complete one of the Part IV MOCA activities through their other certifying Board in substitution for the Part IV: case evaluation requirement [2].

Diplomates Who Are Not Clinically Active

Diplomates who hold time-limited certificates in anesthesiology or a subspecialty but are not clinically active can maintain their certification(s) by participating in the MOCA program [2]. These diplomates are excluded from the Part IV MOCA requirement but must complete all other components of the MOCA program. Diplomates who successfully meet these requirements are designated "Certified—Not Clinically Active." [2].

Diplomates Whose Primary Anesthesiology Certification Has Been Deferred

After passing Parts 1 (written) and 2 (oral) of the initial certification examination, some diplomates may elect to defer primary certification. If certification is deferred for less than 5 years, CME credit earned during the period from completing the oral examination until certification is awarded can be credited toward the Part II: LLSA MOCA requirement. The remainder of the MOCA requirements must be completed within the 10-year time frame [2].

If certification is deferred for more than 5 but less than 10 years, candidates may submit up to 5 years worth of their most current CME credit earned within the years from passing the oral examination until certification is awarded. They have 5 years to complete the remaining MOCA requirements [2].

MOCA Reporting

Although all diplomates are automatically enrolled in the MOCA program upon initial certification, it is the responsibility of diplomates to maintain accurate and up-to-date personal information to the ABA portal.

Furthermore, although some CME sponsors, such as the ASA, the American Society of Regional Anesthesia (ASRA), and the New York State Society of

Anesthesiologists (NYSSA) submit CME activities and credit information directly to the ABA on behalf of diplomates, the majority of CME sponsors do not. Therefore, it is the responsibility of diplomates to self-report CME activities and credits to the ABA electronically through the ABA portal. Whereas provider-reported CME activities are not subject to ABA audit, self-reported CME is; therefore, diplomates are expected to keep documentation of self-reported CME activity for at least 3 years after submission [2].

In 2010, the ABA began publicly reporting the MOCA enrollment status of diplomates through the ABA Diplomate and Candidate Directory and ABA portal. Diplomates are now designated as "meeting MOCA requirements" or "not meeting MOCA requirements." Diplomates are meeting MOCA requirements if their professional standing is satisfactory, and by the end of their fifth MOCA year, they have completed at least half of their CME credits and one Part IV PPAI activity; and by the end of their tenth MOCA year, they have completed all CME credits and two PPAI activities [2]. The Directory also indicates diplomates who are not required to participate in MOCA because they hold non-time-limited certificates [2].

Physicians who have applied for the ABA examination are considered candidates for the ABA examination. The ABA no longer recognizes the term "Board Eligible" as a physician status [2].

Failure to Fulfill MOCA Requirements

For diplomates who hold time-limited certifications, failure to fulfill MOCA requirements at the end of the 10-year cycle results in expiration of ABA certification. The ABA will grant a grace period of up to 3 years in order for a diplomate to regain "Active" status [2]. For each additional year past expiration needed to complete the MOCA requirements, the ABA moves the MOCA cycle forward 1 year, and any activities completed in the original Year 1 of the diplomate's MOCA cycle are erased and must be redone. In addition, any outstanding MOCA activities from the 10-year cycle must be successfully completed [2]. Failure to fulfill MOCA requirements within 3 years of expiration of primary certification requires the diplomate to reestablish qualifications for admission for primary certification, including successful completion of the written and oral ABA Board Examinations. During the grace period, diplomates are not designated as Board certified.

Cost of MOCA

There is a single fee for each 10-year MOCA cycle, due upon registration for the Cognitive Examination. In 2013, the registration fee for the MOCA Cognitive Examination was $2,100; the reexamination fee was $800 [2]. However, this is just a fraction of the complete costs associated with fulfillment of MOCA criteria.

The cost of currently accredited simulation courses is approximately $1,500–$1,800. Although opportunities for free CME credits exist (e.g., Medscape CME), the majority must be purchased. The cost per credit varies widely. For example, for ASA members, the ACE and SEE programs offer CME credit at a rate of $5 per credit. However, the ASA Patient Safety modules run approximately $11 per credit. Factoring in the annual ASA membership due of $625, the relative cost per credit is even higher.

Benefits of MOCA

There is a general perception that having a maintenance of certification (MOC) program helps to ensure the quality of physician care. Indeed, in a 2003 Gallup Poll conducted by the American Board of Internal Medicine, nearly 75 % of respondents agreed with the idea that physicians should be periodically reevaluated on their qualifications, and more than half said they would be inclined to find a new doctor if their current doctor's board certification expired [7]. However, despite its widespread acceptance, that participation in MOC activities actually improves patient outcomes or has a sustained effect on physician decision-making has yet to be demonstrated [8].

Furthermore, there is some evidence to suggest that the physicians who might benefit the most from participation in an MOC program are the very ones who have been given the opportunity to opt out of it altogether. Examining the likelihood of physicians passing a recertification examination in internal medicine, Ramsey and colleagues found a significant inverse relationship between exam scores and number of years since primary certification [9]. Several studies have demonstrated a lower adherence to practice guidelines among older physicians compared to younger colleagues [10–12]. Therefore, the ABA's choice to absolve from MOCA responsibilities diplomates certified prior to 2000 may be considered a missed opportunity.

The ABA's decision to include a simulation course as a MOCA requirement is also controversial. The ABA's support of simulation mirrors that of the Council on Graduate Medical Education and the ABMS, both of which believe that simulation training is an important component of improving patient safety [13]. There is some evidence to support the benefits of simulation relative to traditional learning methods in promoting teamwork and improving performance in critical event management [14, 15]. However, other studies suggest that the same results may be achieved through case-based learning, foregoing the significant expense of a mechanical simulator, which can cost from $6,000 to $250,000 [6, 16]. Although simulation shows promise as an education tool, important questions still remain, including its relative success in changing provider behavior compared to traditional forms of CME, such as classroom learning or workshops [17]. In addition, a link between simulation education and absolute reduction in medical errors or benefit in patient outcomes has yet to be established [18]. While other specialties offer simulation courses, mostly in the form of computerized case-based scenarios, anesthesiology is the only specialty whose MOC program requires diplomates to participate in a hands-on simulation class.

Continual Evolution of MOCA

The MOCA program is a concept in evolution and its requirements are subject to change in response to internal process audits and external governances. It is incumbent on the ABA diplomate to remain vigilant to these changes.

References

1. Rhodes RS, Biester TW. Certification and maintenance of certification in surgery. Surg Clin North Am. 2007;87(4):825–36.
2. American Board of Anesthesiology, Inc. Booklet of information: certification and maintenance of certification. Raleigh, NC: American Board of Anesthesiology, Inc; 2013.
3. American Board of Anesthesiology, Inc. ABA announces 2010 changes to MOCA cognitive examination. ABA News. 2009;22(1):9.
4. American Board of Anesthesiology, Inc. 2011 Examination results. ABA News. pp 31–3.
5. McCarthy JL. An essential tool for patient safety. Forum. 2008;26(4):1–2.
6. Okuda Y, Bryson EO, DeMaria Jr S, Jacobson L, Quinones J, Shen B, et al. The utility of simulation in medical education: what is the evidence? Mt Sinai J Med. 2009;76(4):330–43.
7. The Gallup Organization. Awareness of and attitudes toward board-certification of physicians. Princeton, NJ: The Gallup Organization; 2003.
8. Davis D, O'Brien MA, Freemantle N, Wolf FM, Mazmanian P, Taylor-Vaisey A. Impact of formal continuing medical education: do conferences, workshops, rounds, and other traditional continuing education activities change physician behavior or health care outcomes? JAMA. 1999;282(9):867–74.
9. Ramsey PG, Carline JD, Inui TS, Larson EB, LoGerfo JP, Norcini JJ, et al. Changes over time in the knowledge base of practicing internists. JAMA. 1991;266(8):1103–7.
10. Czaja R, McFall SL, Warnecke RB, Ford L, Kaluzny AD. Preferences of community physicians for cancer screening guidelines. Ann Intern Med. 1994;120(7):602–8.
11. Day SC, Norcini JJ, Webster GD, Viner ED, Chirico AM. The effect of changes in medical knowledge on examination performance at the time of recertification. Res Med Educ. 1988;27:139–44.
12. Eva KW. The aging physician: changes in cognitive processing and their impact on medical practice. Acad Med. 2002;77(10 Suppl):S1–6.
13. ASA Workgroup on Simulation Education. White paper on ASA approval of anesthesiology simulation programs. Raleigh, NC: ASA Workgroup on Simulation Education; 2006.
14. McLaughlin S, Fitch MT, Goyal DG, Hayden E, Kauh CY, Laack TA, et al. Simulation in graduate medical education 2008: a review for emergency medicine. Acad Emerg Med. 2008;15(11):1117–29.
15. Park CS, Rochlen LR, Yaghmour E, Higgins N, Bauchat JR, Wojciechowski KG, et al. Acquisition of critical intraoperative event management skills in novice anesthesiology residents by using high-fidelity simulation-based training. Anesthesiology. 2010;112(1):202–11.
16. Frengley RW, Weller JM, Torrie J, Dzendrowskyj P, Yee B, Paul AM, et al. The effect of a simulation-based training intervention on the performance of established critical care unit teams. Crit Care Med. 2011;39(12):2605–11.

17. Grimshaw JM, Shirran L, Thomas R, Mowatt G, Fraser C, Bero L, et al. Changing provider behavior: an overview of systematic reviews of interventions. Med Care. 2001;39(8 Suppl 2):II2–45.
18. Boulet JR, Murray D. Review article: assessment in anesthesiology education. Can J Anaesth. 2012;59(2):182–92.

Chapter 10
Evaluation of Anesthesiology Residents

John E. Tetzlaff

Abbreviations

ABA	American Board of Anesthesiology
ACGME	Accreditation Council for Graduate Medical Education
AKT	Anesthesia Knowledge Test
AOS	Area of strength
CA-1	Clinical anesthesia, year 1
CA-2	Clinical anesthesia, year 2
CA-3	Clinical anesthesia, year 3
GME	Graduate medical education
ICU	Intensive care unit
ITE	In-training examination
MCQ	Multiple choice question examination
OSCE	Objective structured clinical examination
PACU	Post-anesthesia care unit
PBLI	Practice-based learning and improvement
RIME	"Reporter," "interpreter," "manager," or "educator"
RRC	Residency Review Committee
SP	Standard patient
TAFI	Targeted area for improvement

J.E. Tetzlaff, M.D. (✉)
Cleveland Clinic Lerner College of Medicine,
Case Western Reserve University, Cleveland, OH, USA

Department of General Anesthesia, Anesthesiology Institute,
Cleveland Clinic, 9500 Euclid Avenue, Cleveland, OH 44195, USA
e-mail: tetzlaj@ccf.org

Background

Traditional graduate medical education (GME) has followed the apprenticeship model introduced at the beginning of the twentieth century. After a basic medical education, the resident learned by direct observation of the attending, and evaluation was the converse-direct staff observation of the work or outcome of the work by the resident. This model evolved by the midpoint of the twentieth century to include high-stakes written examinations and specialty certification. In anesthesiology, certification has also included an oral examination. Eligibility for certification starts with the determination by the residency director that the resident is competent. For the majority of the twentieth century, the criteria for competency were completely determined by the individual residency programs. Ultimate certification started with traditional written, multiple choice examinations, graded by standard statistical techniques and concluded with the oral examination, graded in a virtual pass/fail method.

Within residency programs, a variety of evaluation tools were variably deployed. Because of the acute care nature of anesthesia practice, learning of anesthesia techniques by anesthesiology residents occurs under the direct observation of staff during induction, airway management, critical events, and emergence. As a result, evaluations were global ("I know it when I see it") using Likert scales (Table 10.1)

Table 10.1 Sample Likert scale

Staff evaluation of resident professionalism					
Resident name: (picture also)					
Time interval evaluated: (drop down box)					
During this interval, I have not worked with this resident: (check box)					
The resident's conduct within the division is appropriate					
0	**1**	**2**	**3**	**4**	**5**
Not observed	Poor		Good		Excellent
The resident accepts assignment without unreasonable compliant					
0	**1**	**2**	**3**	**4**	**5**
Not observed	Poor		Good		Excellent
Resident interacts appropriately with staff					
0	**1**	**2**	**3**	**4**	**5**
Not observed	Poor		Good		Excellent
Resident interacts with other residents appropriately					
0	**1**	**2**	**3**	**4**	**5**
Not observed	Poor		Good		Excellent
Resident treats patients with respect					
0	**1**	**2**	**3**	**4**	**5**
Not observed	Poor		Good		Excellent
Resident treats nurses with respect					
0	**1**	**2**	**3**	**4**	**5**
Not observed	Poor		Good		Excellent
Resident treats other support personnel with respect					
0	**1**	**2**	**3**	**4**	**5**
Not observed	Poor		Good		Excellent
Comments required for all 1 and 2 responses					

with their known weaknesses [1], based on diversity of cases, didactic teaching, and specialty experience of the staff. Many programs also used measures of medical knowledge from homegrown or standard written examinations ("In-Training Examination" and/or "Anesthesia Knowledge Test"). Even for programs using standard written examinations, the pass/fail criteria and consequences were locally determined. In the latter half of the twentieth century, credit for training by the American Board of Anesthesiology (ABA) was granted in 6-month intervals based on satisfactory reports from Clinical Competence Committees within residency programs, although criteria again were local.

With the approach of the twenty-first century, many forces combined to create a higher level of expectations for outcomes of GME and medicine in general [2]. A major impetus for change came from the federal government, driven by the billions of dollars in direct subsidies of GME from the Medicare program. Similar pressure came from industry and private insurance, where the linkage of quality with cost became increasingly evident. Conditions for participation in many cases have linkage to certification, as well as patient safety initiatives. All have direct implications for GME programs.

Seeing that legislative or administrative rulings would result from failure to act, the Accreditation Council for Graduate Medical Education (ACGME) decided to be proactive and create these rules from within the GME regulatory authority, avoiding the arbitrary and less focused consequences that might have come with governmental action [3]. After an extensive review of existing evaluation techniques within GME funded by the Robert Woods Johnson foundation, the ACGME published six general competencies for all of GME (Table 10.2). Criteria for these competencies were published in 1999 and included a 10-year time line for implementation. Implementation required curricula to establish what was being taught for each competency as well as how it would be assessed. General criteria for all GME programs were supplemented by specialty-specific criteria dictated by the Residency Review Committee (RRC) within the ACGME for each specialty. Evaluation has evolved toward "assessment of competence," which shortens to assessment. The final upcoming element for assessment of competencies is the Milestones Project of the ACGME, in which specialty-specific performance criteria must be established and promotion tied to achievement of these goals as opposed to time limits.

Assessment Versus Evaluation

The element of an intervention that distinguishes it as assessment is the desire to select a tool that is consistent, reliable, and based on objective criteria [4]. The goal of the intervention is also important, as there are both "formative" assessment and "summative" assessment [5]. Formative assessment is a collection of information about a resident, usually behavioral, designed as feedback to drive learning. The emphasis of formative assessment is the use of multiple tools and multiple sources of assessment. The stakes for any given formative assessment are low enough that the student can accept the content in the spirit of targeted areas for improvement (TAFI).

Table 10.2 ACGME general competencies

1. *Patient care*: The residency program must ensure that its residents, by the time they graduate, provide appropriate, effective, and compassionate clinical care. Residents are expected to:
   - Communicate effectively and demonstrate caring and respectful behaviors when interacting with patients and patients' families
   - Gather essential and accurate information about the patient and use it together with up-to-date scientific evidence to make decisions about diagnostic and therapeutic interventions
   - Develop and carry out patient management plans
   - Provide education and counseling to patients
   - Perform competently all medical and invasive procedures essential for the area of practice
   - Provide health care services aimed at preventing health problems or maintaining health
   - Work with other health care professionals to provide patient-focused care
2. *Medical knowledge*: The residency program must ensure that its residents, by the time they graduate, possess knowledge in established and evolving biomedical and clinical science domains and apply it to clinical care Residents are expected to:
   - Demonstrate rigor in their thinking about clinical situations
   - Know and apply the basic and clinically supportive sciences which are appropriate to their discipline
3. *Practice-based learning and improvement*: The residency program must ensure that its residents, by the time they graduate, are able to investigate, evaluate, and improve their patient care practices. Residents are expected to:
   - Analyze practice experience and perform practice-based improvement activities using systematic methodology
   - Locate, appraise, and assimilate "best practices" related to their patients' health problems
   - Apply knowledge of study designs and statistical methods to the appraisal of clinical studies and other information on diagnostic and therapeutic effectiveness
   - Use information technology to manage information; access online medical information; and support clinical care, patient education, and their own education
4. *Interpersonal and communication skills*: The residency program must ensure that its residents, by the time they graduate, can develop appropriate interpersonal relationships and communicate effectively with patients, their patient's families, and professional associates. Residents are expected to:
   - Create and sustain a therapeutic and ethically sound relationship with patients
   - Elicit and provide information using effective nonverbal, explanatory, questioning, and writing skills
   - Work effectively with others as a member or leader of a professional group, in particular a health care team that might include professionals from other disciplines
5. *Professionalism*: The residency program must ensure that its residents, by the time they graduate, demonstrate the fundamental qualities of professionalism. Residents are expected to:
   - Demonstrate respect, regard, integrity, and a responsiveness to the needs of patients and society that supercedes self-interest; assume responsibility and act responsibly; and demonstrate a commitment to excellence and ongoing professional development
   - Demonstrate a commitment to ethical principles pertaining to the provision or withholding of clinical care, confidentiality of patient information, informed consent, and business practices demonstrate sensitivity and responsiveness to cultural differences, including awareness of their own and patients' cultural perspectives

(continued)

Table 10.2 (continued)

6. *Systems-based practice*: The residency program must ensure that its residents, by the time they graduate, are aware that health care is provided in the context of a larger system and can effectively call on the system resources to support the care of patients. Residents are expected to:
 - Understand how their patient care practices and related actions impact component units of the health care delivery system and the total delivery system and how delivery systems impact the provision of health care
 - Know systems-based approaches for controlling health care costs and allocating resources and practice cost-effective health care and resource allocation that does not compromise quality of care
 - Advocate for quality patient care and assist patients in dealing with system complexities
 - Know how to partner with health care managers and health care providers to assess, coordinate, and improve health care and know how these activities can impact system

Formative assessment is usually balanced, and areas of strength (AOS) are delivered with the same level of importance as TAFI. With multiple assessments over the same time interval (or rotation), the significance of any one assessment is not excessive, and the outcome is determined by the overall impression obtained from all the evaluations. Such a practice decreases the importance of any one tool. Moreover it allows some freedom for various tools to be applied to any given assessment interval.

While formative assessment is becoming more universal in GME, the tradition has been "high-stakes" or summative assessment. These actions are usually single events with a tool selected for various reasons including expedience and tradition. Examples include the global rotation assessment for clinical skills and the written, multiple choice in-training examinations for medical knowledge, as well as the 6 month report of the Clinical Competence Committee. The summative assessment is associated with a consequence (pass/fail, promotion, etc.) which attaches a high level of significance to both the program and the student. Since it is often a single event, the appropriateness of the tool to measure the intended target is high. The pressure of the event also has consequences, because the student is aware of the high level of significance of the summative assessment and directs a high level of attention ("study to the test") to the summative event and to the detriment of other learning opportunities. In the case of the high-stakes written examination, there is intense studying immediately prior to the event, followed by limited retention after the event ("binge and purge"), ultimately with limited learning [6]. The anxiety created by the "study-test" cycle actually opposes learning [7]. The impact on the program can also be an emphasis in the curriculum on the cyclic occurrence of the in-training examination [8].

An appropriate approach to overall assessment should include a balance of formative and summative assessments, and the tools selected for each assessment should be chosen because they measure what is intended [9]. As an example, the United States Medical Licensing Examinations (USMLE) are widely recognized as a valid assessment of the breadth of medical knowledge [10]. By extension, the Anesthesiology In-Training Examination (ITE) and the ABA Part 1 examination have the same validity for measurement of medical knowledge. It is less clear, however, if standard written examinations can be used to measure clinical performance for anesthesiology residents. Although there is general evidence that written examinations predict clinical performance for fully trained physicians in the practice [11], the evidence for residents is contradictory. In one report, an effort to predict critical incidents from review of written examination showed no correlation with actual clinical outcomes for the same residents [12]. The written examination reliably measures the medical knowledge tested, but less reliably predicts higher cognitive functions such as correlation skills and problem solving [13]. The split between assessment of breadth of knowledge and clinical performance is also manifest on the program side. Faculty who have direct knowledge of the clinical performance of a resident [14] may not be accurate in predicting the ITE scores of the same resident [15]. When multiple assessments with good reliability create different results for a resident, the conclusion drawn is that they measure different elements of performance, arguing for the value of multiple tool assessment [16].

Selecting Assessment Tools for Anesthesiology Residents

The optimum strategy for assessment should involve an approach that places emphasis on learning, influenced by content, format, focus, and frequency. Assessment that encourages learning involves feedback to the learner (TAFI and AOS) temporally proximate to the assessment event. This is the time when the learner is most motivated to use feedback to improve performance. Ideal performance feedback should be real time, directly creating learning energy proximate to the event. Interestingly, feedback also improves teaching by faculty [17].

Individual assessment tools should be selected based on their performance for six standard criteria [8]. *Reliability* is the ability of the tool to repeatedly produce the same outcome. It is the consistency, generalizability, or reproducibility of a given tool. If a tool is used by two different faculty members, both should independently arrive at the same conclusion if the tool is reliable. For this criterion, the ITE is excellent. Unstructured global assessment of resident performance has a less favorable reliability factor. *Validity* is the ability of a given assessment tool to measure what it is chosen to measure. Validity is best evident when there is specific measurement in a specific situation in a homogenous group of individuals. While written examinations have good validity for measurement of the breadth of knowledge, they are less valid for the assessment of patient care and clinical skills. Global assessments of clinical procedures have good validity when performed in real time with the clinical event, with validity decreasing with time, and very little validity after 10–14 days [18]. When documentation is delayed, the assessment loses value as a learning experience and may be subject to grading inflation and bias [6]. *Comprehensiveness* is the ability of a given assessment tool to measure all elements of performance in a given epoch of time. Global rotation assessments and objective structured clinical examinations (OSCE) score high in this criterion, where multiple choice examinations are poor choices for comprehensiveness. *Feasibility* is the ability of a given assessment tool to be applied to a specific element of a training program. Direct observation of procedural skill is very feasible in procedure-based specialties (e.g., anesthesiology), where it has lower feasibility in the cognitive-based primary care specialties where the number of repetitions of procedures is less. *Flexibility* is the option to use the tool in a variety of settings. The oral examination format can be adapted to a wide variety of clinical scenarios and, as such, has a high range of flexibility. An OSCE setting can also be adapted to some degree and has reasonable flexibility. A multiple choice standard examination only applies to the setting where it is deployed and as such has limited flexibility. *Accountability* is the ability to defend the efficacy of an assessment tool. A standardized written examination can be evaluated statistically, and the accuracy of the distinction between good performance and poor performance can be determined with a high degree of certainty. As such, the multiple choice questions (MCQ) exam has a high level of accountability for the measurement of the breadth of medical knowledge. A global assessment of a rotation lacks the ability to evaluate the assessment and, as such, has a lower level of accountability.

Assessment of Competence

One of the ways to move from traditional evaluation of resident performance (global rotation score, written in-training examination) to a fuller assessment is to move toward tools that are descriptive. One of the approaches that has been used for medical students includes the sequential descriptors of "reporter," "interpreter," "manager," or "educator" (RIME) indicating progressively more competency as the behavioral terms are met [19]. The Outcomes Project of the Accreditation Council for Graduate Medical Education (ACGME) defined six core competencies that are defined descriptively, including patient care, medical knowledge, interpersonal and communication skills, professionalism, practice-based learning and improvement (PBLI), and systems-based practice. There is evidence that optimum methods of assessing competency for medical knowledge [20], professionalism [21], and patient care [22] involve detecting gaps in performance with descriptive assessment. With assessment of competence, each individual assessment is not as important as the sum of the total assessment, with more assessments being better. With multiple assessments, there is the opportunity to measure competencies for the same variable over time, increasing validity [23]. Another attractive opportunity with multiple assessments is the ability to create an assessment profile for each individual, eliminating the need to consider "strict" or "easy" graders [24].

Assessment Tools for Anesthesiology Residency

There are a wide variety of options for assessment of competencies of anesthesiology residency. In order for the goal of promotion of learning to be achieved, the assessment tool should be selected to fit the learning environment and delivered in a time frame that optimizes the assessment as well as the encouragement of learning. Clearly, the assessment plan should be tailored to fit the teaching style (didactic and clinical) with a mixture of formative (the majority) and summative (only as much as needed) assessments, performed over time. The tools selected need to be varied across the learning domains, since different assessment approaches for technical, cognitive, and behavioral competencies are required [25]. Much is known about each of the individual tools, including characteristics as well as the applicability to individual competencies.

Audits

The combination of guided review of medical records combined with direct feedback to the learner makes the audit technique valuable for assessment of elements of patient care, professionalism, and problem-based learning initiative (PBLI). In general terms, auditing of medical practice can encourage completeness and preferred clinical behavior [26]. Within anesthesiology, general auditing may have limited return for considerable effort because of the structural repetitiveness between cases. However, auditing can be applied to elements of professionalism and PBLI, including data needed for billing and reconciliation of controlled substances with appropriate assessment value for the effort expended.

Direct Observation

Direct observation is undoubtedly the most common assessment tool deployed during anesthesiology residency. Because of the acute care nature of the field, there is daily opportunity for direct observation of clinical performance with the optimum characteristic of being able to make the same observation over time. In general, direct observation is more valid when structured [27]. When structured observation is compared to unstructured observation, it is clear that the faculty miss the extremes of good and bad performance when the observation is unstructured [28, 29]. Structured observation is achieved by behaviorally structured goals and objectives for clinical rotations that are created by the faculty performing the assessments. Although not practical in most residency programs, direct observation improves as an assessment tool when the observer is not involved in the clinical care provided by the learner [30]. Another element that improves the quality of the assessment during direct observation is a checklist, applied uniformly for all learners being assessed in the same setting. A sample checklist that could be used for assessment during direct observation is found in Table 10.3.

Table 10.3 Sample checklist

Assessment of informed consent by anesthesiology resident (yes/no)
1. Identifies self, including residency status (Y/N)
2. Uses appropriate information to identify patient (Y/N)
3. Confirms the correct procedure (Y/N)
4. Confirms correct side (Y/N)
5. Confirms NPO status (Y/N)
6. Explains anesthetic options (Y/N)
7. Asks if surgeon has identified a preference (Y/N)
8. Presents a reasonable list of risks, benefits, and options (Y/N)
9. Answers questions (Y/N)
10. Confirms a choice (Y/N)
11. Confirms that patient is willing to proceed (Y/N)
Number correct:_____

Mentorship

For the behavioral competencies, especially PBLI, mentorship has a role in teaching as well as assessment. The learner has a clinical experience and, shortly after, shares this experience with a senior clinician who provides feedback and TAFI [31]. The role of mentorship within anesthesiology residency setting is best evident in the use of simulation with defined scenarios, experienced and then de-briefed for the learner. Use of evidence-based medicine in clinical care is encouraged by mentorship interactions.

Objective Structured Clinical Examination

The versatility of the OSCE as an assessment tool has received wide recognition for undergraduate and primary care GME programs. Usually involving standardized patients (SP), the OSCE can be created to fit the learning environment and across specialties. The goals of real-time learning from assessment can be achieved, as most OSCE designs include direct feedback immediately after the simulated clinical experience. The role of SP favors the primary care specialties and group who work in medical school setting, due to the demands for recruitment and training of the SP. The OSCE format has been modified to assessment of technical skills and when combined with simulation can assess skills with bronchoscopy, endoscopy, laparoscopy, airway management, and acute care problem solving skills [32, 33]. Because recruitment of standardized patients is not ideally suited to anesthesiology residency, the OSCE format has not been widely adopted within anesthesiology [34], although a simulation-based OSCE has been added to a certification examination setting [35]. Variations on the OSCE theme, including case presentation and the communication elements of the oral exam, have been used for the assessment of the communications competency.

Oral Examination

Anesthesiology is one of the minority of specialties that includes an oral examination as an element of board certification. As such, it is common for the anesthesiology resident to experience one or more oral examinations as part of the core residency. Some programs use the oral examination for formative feedback about breadth of knowledge and/or exam taking skills [36]. Others use the oral examination for summative assessment, with or without feedback about performance. The guided-question format creates some standardization for the learner experience within a group. Validity is improved with repetition by the resident and with faculty training [37]. There is universal agreement that the oral examination format provides valid assessment of the depth of medical knowledge and is a better predictor of clinical decision making, as compared to the written examination format [38]. A promising area for future development is the use of the oral exam format to make assessment of communication skills.

Peer Review

Undergraduate medical education environments are increasingly recognizing the value of peer review assessment [39], especially for the behavioral competencies (professionalism, communications). Primary care GME programs are using the 360° review which includes peer review evidence [40]. Pure peer review has limited application within anesthesiology because of the limited number of settings where team care is provided. However, in defined settings, the limited 360° review ("snapshot") is possible when anesthesiology residents are assigned to the post-anesthesia care unit (PACU), intensive care unit (ICU), and chronic pain clinic. This appraisal can include peer review. Another element of peer review can come from anonymous assessment of professionalism by chief residents, based on their interactions with didactics, call schedules, etc. In a variation to the peer review theme, group project development has demonstrated efficacy for learning and assessment of systems-based practice within an anesthesiology residency [41].

Portfolio Assessment

The use of portfolio creation as an assessment tool originates from the graphic arts and has been widely applied within schools of education. There has been some progress in the deployment of portfolio systems for all or part of the assessment process in medical schools in the United States, the United Kingdom, and Europe. An attractive element of portfolio assessment is the shift of responsibility from the program to the learner. In portfolio assessment, the learner is obligated to actively seek assessment, and the response of the faculty is tracked. The movement of portfolio assessment into GME seems inevitable with the introduction of the ACGME Outcomes Project. The starting point for portfolio assessment is the definition of competencies and the six core competencies of the Outcomes Project are ideally suited to portfolio assessment. The next step is the definition of behaviorally based standards that can be used to determine whether the learner has achieved satisfactory performance in each of the competencies [42]. Standards for competencies are found in the Outcomes Project, with each competencies being defined by its standards. The challenging part is identifying the evidence to be used, comprehensively collecting the evidence and creating a standardized approach to assessment of the evidence [43]. Portfolio assessment could be applied to one, several, or all the competencies. The portfolio review would determine if the resident has met the standards or did not meet or did not provide enough evidence. This is where the reversal of responsibility is most evident. If this system is adopted, the creation of the portfolio is the responsibility of the resident, as is the collection of evidence [44], which inherently involves practice-based learning. An additional advantage is the reflection required by the resident to create the portfolio and the learning that results from the reflection [13], although there is evidence that reflection will not spontaneously occur unless encouraged in anesthesiology residents [45]. Of course, this result is only possible with high level buy-in from the program and the entire faculty, because the resident must be able to ask for evidence (multiple formative assessments), which must be provided in useful format in a timely manner [46]. The feasibility is greatly enhanced when electronic evidence management is developed [47]. Paper-based portfolio, even limited exercises, is difficult to manage, physically large, and hard to maintain.

Self-Assessment

If the goal of learning from assessment is considered, self-assessment is a highly attractive choice. Perhaps because this has not been common in GME, there are limited reports of self-assessment in this setting, although it has increasing use within the undergraduate medical education world. Where it has been reported, with relatively little training, residents have been able to achieve the same assessment of themselves as their faculty. This finding contrasts with self-assessment by physicians in practice, where very limited correlation was found, and an inverse relationship was found in those with least skills [48, 49]. A training effect may be evident in the good correlation by residents after repetition. When self-assessment is combined with auditing, residents can form learning plans to address gaps in their knowledge or missing technical skills. One additional advantage to self-assessment is that when a gap in knowledge is identified, it encourages learning in this element. Self-reporting of medical errors has been reported within anesthesiology, with good potential for learning from experience. The mortality and morbidity conference presentation is another excellent example of learning by self-reporting. When presented with simulated crisis scenario, the self-assessment of performance by the anesthesiology resident was equally effective compared to trained instructors [50]. In another setting for simulation-based self-assessment, trainees with the lower levels of performance consistently overrated their own performance [51]. Self-assessment is part of the continuous quality improvement processes that are part of virtually every anesthesia department and can easily be modified to assessment of resident performance as an element of PBLI.

Simulation

As an alternative to the feasibility issues with OSCE and SP, anesthesiology has widely embraced the learning and assessment opportunities with simulation. There is some evidence that there is adequate reliability and validity in well-designed simulation setting to allow summative assessment [52], even for senior residents as validated by other assessments tools [53]. Full-scale human patient simulation has been used to teach and assess airway skill in novices, hemodynamic manipulation, as well as management of uncommon clinical crises, similar to the de-briefing of "near-misses" in the aviation industry [54–57]. For anesthesiology residents, simulation-based skill assessment demonstrated good efficacy to distinguish the skill set of experienced residents compared to beginners [58, 59]. These exercises include technical as well as nontechnical skills [60]. The assessment opportunity is the ability to define behavioral responses to critical incidents, such as machine failure, in a simulated environment for anesthesiology residents [61]. In the surgical world, simulated performance of tasks such as endoscopy or laparoscopy correlated very well with the assessment of the resident's skills in the operating room. Some skills require only instruction and the opportunity to practice on a mannequin, prior to achieving satisfactory performance [62]. Simulation could also be used as an adjunct to oral examination of senior residents and may detect gaps in clinical skill not detected by the oral examination format [63]. Simulation also presents the opportunity to assess the performance of anesthesiology residents for rare critical events, not often encountered in the operating room [64]. It has been used to evaluate the validity of other assessment tools used within anesthesiology residency [65].

Standardized Patients

The use of standardized patients has achieved wide acceptance for assessment of clinical skills and clinical reasoning of medical students [25]. The feasibility issues with SP have been previously discussed, and one additional issue is the demand on faculty for recruitment and training of SP. While SP experiences provide good assessment for novices, their value decreases with experience, as the opportunity to detect gaps in knowledge becomes less robust with senior trainees [25]. As previously mentioned, SP use within anesthesiology has not achieved widespread application because anesthesiology practice does not lend itself well to the recruitment of SP. Limited use for the testing of communication skills or the ability to teach and assess the resident ability to deliver bad news is a potential avenue for the inroad of SP into anesthesiology residency.

Written Examination

Written (now electronic) MCQ examinations have wide recognition for the ability to define the breadth of medical knowledge. It is less clear that they define skill with patient care and have limited, if any role, in the assessment of behavioral competencies [5]. The extended match format has been added to written examinations to expand the ability to assess patient care skills. When traditional MCQ is compared to other assessment tools, such as OSCE or extended match questions in medical students, the results make it clear that each tool is measuring a different domain of knowledge. Another important element of the high-stakes MCQ examination is the impact on learning. There is intense studying immediately prior to the exam ("cramming") followed by considerable loss of knowledge ("binge and purge") in the aftermath [8]. It is equally clear that placing emphasis on the written examination alters the didactic curriculum ("studying to the test") in a manner not optimum for long-term learning. The role of the written examination has a traditional place within anesthesiology. Virtually all programs require their residents to take the annual in-training examination and use the results for formative assessment and remediation based on reported keywords where a majority have answered incorrectly. Some programs use the exam in part for summative assessment, including promotion decisions. Some programs use the additional information obtained from the independent Anesthesia Knowledge Test (AKT) which can be administered at 1, 6, and 18 months. Written examinations within anesthesiology are acknowledged to measure breadth of knowledge, although not necessarily depth of knowledge. Thus, the oral examination remains part of the ABA certification process. And errors in a written examination format do not necessarily correlate with unsatisfactory clinical performance [12]. On the other hand, written examinations do predict performance on other standardized examinations [66] and may predict overall performance during GME [67].

The Next Accreditation System: The Anesthesiology Milestones

One tradition for GME has been the separation of residents by year groups and promotion based on the calendar (first year, second year, etc.). While this has also been linked to achievement of defined goals (ITE, number of cases, specific rotations, etc.), it is also at least partly chronological. With the creation of the Next

Accreditation System (NAS) by the ACGME, each specialty will be tasked to develop performance criteria for competencies (milestones) and assess the resident based on achievement of competencies instead of time in the program [68]. As opposed to clinical base year, clinical anesthesia-year 1, 2, or 3 (CA-1, CA-2, and CA-3), the knowledge and skills will be defined as entry level (end of clinical base year), junior level (end of CA-1 year), mid-level (after subspecialty rotations), senior level (ready to graduate), and advanced level. For each competency, specialty-specific skills will be defined and descriptive standards created to define each level. A preliminary draft of the anesthesia milestones reveals variability in the number of standards within each competency, with the largest number (not surprisingly) being with the patient care competency. The level of supervision by staff is also defined by direct supervision, indirect supervision, and oversight. The goal over time is to define the resident participation in the training program by acquired skill and knowledge as opposed to appointment year level. What is left to the program as a challenge for the upcoming decade is to identify the kind of evidence that will be used to determine if the resident has achieved the standards of the competencies ("milestone").

Obstacles to Overcome to Achieve Effective Assessment of Residents

The greatest single barrier to improve assessment of the competency of anesthesiology residents are the habits formed over years of GME experience, dating from when the program director and faculty were residents themselves. It is easy to depend on the score of a written examination and equally easy to define the resident based on a single experience ("I know it when I see it"). Although the education literature clearly establishes that "studying to the test" is the enemy of learning, didactic curriculum continue to be designed to improve test scores [8]. It is equally true that the education literature supports the efficacy of multiple tools to evaluate performance, but habit leads to the use of a single tool (global rotation assessment) to define performance. Rotation assessments suffer from the known limitation of the Likert scales and the "halo" effect, where the outcome is determined by what is known to have occurred in the past. Just exposure to good performance led faculty to rate borderline performance of other performers lower than those faculty not preconditioned by experience with superior performers [69]. There are "tough graders," "down the middle," and the "easy grader" with grade inflation occurring in all of these categories, unless each faculty is evaluated and given a normal range, allowing the opportunity to predict individual residency performance over time and compared to others [24]. And much of what is taught in residency programs is not directly in the curriculum ("hidden curriculum"). Finally, there has never been a systematic approach to evaluating assessment determinations as they influence the education outcome, i.e., assessment of competence of graduates of the training program.

A systematic review of the self-assessment of graduates of a training program would provide interesting insight for those in charge of the curriculum and assessment process [70].

References

1. Loyd GE, Koenig HM. Assessment of learning outcomes. Summative evaluations. Int Anesthesiol Clin. 2008;46:97–111.
2. Glance LG, Neuman M, Martinez EA, Pauker KY, Dutton RP. Performance measures at a "tipping point". Anesth Analg. 2011;112:958–66.
3. Accreditation Council for Graduate Medical Education. Common program requirements: general competencies. http://www.acgme.org/acgmeweb/Portals/0/PFAssets/ProgramRequirements/CPRs2013.pdf. Accessed 23 Sep 2013.
4. Pangaro L. A new vocabulary and other innovations for improving descriptive in-training evaluations. Acad Med. 1999;74:1203–7.
5. Tetzlaff JE. Assessment of competence in anesthesiology. Anesthesiology. 2007;106:812–25.
6. Turnbull J, Gray J, MacFadyen J. Improving in-training evaluation programs. J Gen Intern Med. 1998;13:317–23.
7. De Oliveira Filho GR, Vieira JE. The relationship of learning environment, quality of life, and study strategies measures to anesthesiology resident academic performance. Anesth Analg. 2007;104:1467–72.
8. Shumway JM, Harden RM. AMEE guide no. 25: The assessment of learning outcomes for the competent and reflective physician. Med Teach. 2003;25:569–84.
9. Friedman Ben-David M. AMEE guide no. 14: outcome-based education: part 3—assessment in outcome-based education. Med Teach. 1999;21:121–3.
10. Williams III RG. Use of NBME and USMLE examinations to evaluate medical education programs. Acad Med. 1993;68:748–52.
11. Norcini JJ, Swanson DB, Grosso LF, Shea JA, Webster GD. A comparison of knowledge, synthesis and clinical judgment: multiple choice questions in the assessment of physician competence. Eval Health Prof. 1984;7:485–500.
12. Slogoff S, Hughes FP. Validity of scoring "dangerous answers" on a written certification examination. J Med Educ. 1987;62:625–31.
13. Friedman Ben-David M. The role of assessment in expanding professional horizons. Med Teach. 2000;22:9–16.
14. Hawkins RE, Sumption KF, Gaglione MM, Holmbor ES. The in training examination in internal medicine: resident perceptions and the lack of correlation between resident score and faculty prediction of resident performance. Am J Med. 1999;106:206–10.
15. Wise S, Stagg L, Szucs R, Gay S, Mauger D, Hartman D. Assessment of resident knowledge: subjective assessment versus performance on the ACR in-training examination. Acad Radiol. 1999;6:66–71.
16. Schwartz RW, Donnelly MB, Sloan DA, Johnson SB, Strodel WE. Assessing senior residents' knowledge and performance: an integrated evaluation program. Surgery. 1994;116:634–40.
17. Baker K. Clinical teaching improves with resident evaluation and feedback. Anesthesiology. 2010;113:693–703.
18. Norman GR, van der Vleuten CPM, de Graffe E. Pitfalls in the pursuit of objectivity: issues of validity, efficiency and acceptability. Med Educ. 1991;25:119–26.
19. Pangaro LN. Investing in descriptive evaluation: a vision for the future of assessment. Med Teach. 2000;22:478–81.
20. Hemmer PA, Pangaro LN. The effect of formal evaluation sessions during clinical clerkships in better identifying students with marginal fund of knowledge. Acad Med. 1997;72:641–3.

21. Hemmer PA, Hawkins R, Jackson JL, Pangaro LN. Assessing how well three evaluation methods detect deficiencies in medical students' professionalism in two settings of an internal medicine clerkship. Acad Med. 2000;75:167–73.
22. Lavin B, Pangaro LN. Internship ratings as a validity measure for an evaluation system to identify inadequate clerkship performance. Acad Med. 1998;75:998–1002.
23. Rose SH, Burkle CM. Accreditation Council for Graduate Medical Education competencies and the American Board of Anesthesiology Clinical Competence Committee: a comparison. Anesth Analg. 2006;102:212–6.
24. Baker K. Determining resident performance. Getting beyond the noise. Anesthesiology. 2011;115:862–78.
25. Tetzlaff JE. Assessment of competence in anesthesiology. Curr Opin Anaesthesiol. 2009;22:809–13.
26. Wainwright JR, Sullivan FM, Morrison JM, MacNaughton RJ, McConnadrie A. Audit encourages an evidence-based approach to medical practice. Med Educ. 1999;33:907–14.
27. Epstein RM. Assessment in medical education. N Engl J Med. 2007;356:387–96.
28. Noel G, Herbers J, Caplow M, Cooper G, Pangaro L, Harvey J. How well do internal medicine faculty members evaluate the clinical skills of residents? Ann Intern Med. 1992;117(9):757–65.
29. Herberts J, Gordon N, Cooper G, Harvey J, Pangaro L, Weaver M. How accurate are faculty evaluations of clinical competence? J Gen Intern Med. 1989;4:202–8.
30. Cydulka RK, Emerman CL, Jouriles NJ. Evaluation of resident performance and intensive bedside teaching during direct observation. Acad Emerg Med. 1996;3:345–51.
31. Connor MP, Bynoe AG, Redfern N, Pokora J, Clarke J. Developing senior doctors as mentors: a form of continuing professional development. Report of an initiative to develop a network of senior doctors as mentors: 1994–99. Med Educ. 2000;34:747–53.
32. MacRae H, Regehr G, Leadbetter W, Reznick R. A comprehensive examination for senior surgery residents. Am J Surg. 2000;179:190–3.
33. Bann S, Datta V, Khan M, Darzi A. The surgical error examination is a novel method for objective technical knowledge assessment. Am J Surg. 2003;185(6):507–11.
34. Boulet JR, Murray D, Kras J, Woodhouse J, McAllister J, Ziv A. Reliability and validity of a simulation-based acute care skills assessment for medical students and residents. Anesthesiology. 2003;99(6):1270–80.
35. Berkenstadt H, Ziv A, Gafni N, Sidi A. Incorporating simulation-based objective structured clinical examination into the Israeli national board examination in anesthesiology. Anesth Analg. 2006;102:853–8.
36. Schubert A, Tetzlaff JE, Licina M, Mascha E, Smith MP. Organization of a comprehensive anesthesiology oral practice examination program: planning, structure, startup, administration, growth and evaluation. J Clin Anesth. 1999;11:504–18.
37. Jacobsohn E, Klock PA, Avidan M. Poor inter-rater reliability on mock anesthesia oral examinations. Can J Anaesth. 2006;53:659–68.
38. Eagle CJ, Martineau R, Hamilton K. The oral examination in anesthetic resident evaluation. Can J Anaesth. 1993;40:947–53.
39. Dannefer EF, Henson LC, Bierer SB, Grady-Weliky TA, Meldrum S, Nofziger AC, Barclay C, Epstein RM. Peer assessment of professional competence. Med Educ. 2005;39:713–22.
40. Ramsey PG, Wenrich MD, Carline JD, et al. Use of peer ratings to evaluate physician performance. JAMA. 1993;269:1655–60.
41. Delphin E, Davidson M. Teaching and evaluating group competency in systems-based practice in anesthesiology. Anesth Analg. 2008;106:1837–43.
42. O'Sullivan PS, Cogbill KK, McClain T, Reckase MD, Clardy JA. Portfolios as a novel approach for residency evaluation. Acad Psychiatry. 2002;26:173–9.
43. Friedman Ben-David M, Davis MH, Harden RM, Howie PW, Ker J, Pippard MJ. AMEE medical education guide no. 24: portfolios as a method of student assessment. Med Teach. 2001;23:535–51.
44. O'Sullivan P, Greene C. Portfolios: possibilities for addressing emergency medicine resident competencies. Acad Emerg Med. 2002;9:1305–9.

45. Houben KW, van den Hombergh CLM, Stalmeijer RE, Scherpbier AJ, Marcus MAE. New training strategies for anaesthesia residents. Curr Opin Anaesthesiol. 2011;24:682–6.
46. Driessen EW, van Tartwijk J, Overeem K, Vermunt JD, van der Vleuten CPM. Conditions for successful reflective use of portfolios in undergraduate medical education. Med Educ. 2005;39:1230–5.
47. Parboosingh J. Learning portfolios: potential to assist health professionals with self-directed learning. J Contin Educ Health Prof. 1996;16:75–81.
48. Davis DA, Mazmanian PE, Fordis M, Harrison RV, Thorpe KE, Perrier L. Accuracy of physician self-assessment compared with observed measures of competence: a systematic review. JAMA. 2006;296:1094–102.
49. Schartel SA, Metro DG. Evaluation: measuring performance, ensuring competence, achieving long-term excellence. Anesthesiology. 2010;112:519–20.
50. Boet S, Bould MD, Bruppacher HR, Desjardins F, Chandra DB, Naik VN. Looking in the mirror: self-debriefing versus instructor debriefing for simulated crises. Crit Care Med. 2011;39:1377–81.
51. Weller JM, Robinson BJ, Jolly B, Watterson LM, Joseph M, Bajenov S, Haughton AJ, Larsen PD. Psychometric characteristics of simulation-based assessment in anaesthesia and accuracy of self-assessed score. Anaesthesia. 2005;60:245–50.
52. LeBlanc VR. Review article: simulation in anesthesia: state of the science and looking forward. Can J Anaesth. 2012;59:193–202.
53. Mudumbai SC, Gaba DM, Boulet JR, Howard SK, Davies MF. External validation of simulation-based assessment with other performance measures of third-year anesthesiology residents. Simul Healthc. 2012;7:73–80.
54. Gaba DM, Howard SK, Flanagan B, Smith BE, Fish KJ, Botney R. Assessment of clinical performance during simulated crises using both technical and behavioral ratings. Anesthesiology. 1998;89(1):8–18.
55. Murray DJ, Boulet JR, Kras JF, Woodhouse JA, Cox T, McAllister JD. Acute care skills in anesthesia practice: a simulation-based resident performance assessment. Anesthesiology. 2004;101(5):1084–95.
56. Schwid HA, Rooke GA, Carline J, Steadman RH, Murray WB, Olympio M, Tarver S, Steckner K, Wetstone S; Anesthesia Simulator Research Consortium. Evaluation of anesthesia residents using mannequin-based simulation: a multi-institutional study. Anesthesiology. 2002;97(6):1434–44.
57. Helmreich RL, Davies JM. Anaesthetic simulation and lessons to be learned from aviation. Can J Anaesth. 1997;44:907–12.
58. Murray DJ, Boulet JR, Avidan M, Kras JF, Henrichs D, Woodhouse J. Performance of residents and anesthesiologists in a simulation-based skill assessment. Anesthesiology. 2007;107:705–13.
59. Fehr JJ, Boulet JR, Waldrop WB, Snider R, Brockel M, Murray DJ. Simulation-based assessment of pediatric anesthesia skills. Anesthesiology. 2011;115:1308–15.
60. Boulet JR, Murray D. Review article: assessment in anesthesiology education. Can J Anaesth. 2012;59:182–92.
61. Waldrop WB, Murray DJ, Boulet JR, Kras JF. Management of anesthesia equipment failure: a simulation-based resident skill assessment. Anesth Analg. 2009;109:426–33.
62. Pott LM, Santrock D. Teaching without a teacher: developing competencies with a Bullard laryngoscope using only a structured self-learning course and practicing on a mannequin. J Clin Anesth. 2007;19:583–6.
63. Savoldelli GL, Naik VN, Joo HS, Houston PL, Graham M, Yee B, Hamstra SJ. Evaluation of patient simulator performance as an adjunct to the oral examination for senior anesthesia residents. Anesthesiology. 2006;104:475–81.
64. Gallagher CJ, Tan JM. The current status of simulation in the maintenance of certification. Int Anesthesiol Clin. 2010;48:83–99.
65. Steadman RH, Huang YM. Simulation for quality assurance in training, credentialing and maintenance of certification. Best Pract Res Clin Anaesthesiol. 2012;26:3–15.

66. Kearney RA, Sullivan P, Skakun E. Performance on ABA-ASA in-training examination predicts success for RCPSC certification. Can J Anaesth. 2000;47:914–8.
67. Berner ES, Brooks CM, Erdmann IV JB. Use of the USMLE to select residents. Acad Med. 1993;68:753–9.
68. Nasca TJ, Philibert I, Brigham T, Flynn TC. The next GME accreditation system—rationale and benefits. N Engl J Med. 2012;366:1051–6.
69. Yeates P, O'Neill P, Mann K, Eva KW. Effect of exposure to good versus poor medical trainee performance on attending physician ratings of subsequent performances. JAMA. 2012;308: 2226–32.
70. Asch DA, Epstein A, Nicholson S. Evaluating medical training programs by the quality of care delivered by their alumni. JAMA. 2007;298:1049–51.

Chapter 11
Giving Feedback to Superiors-Attending Evaluation

Shara Steiner Brody, Julie Oppenheimer, and Michael C. Lewis

Why Is It Important to Give Feedback?

It's well known that in the context of graduate medical education (GME) giving feedback is a skill that is challenging and rewarding for both the teacher (e.g., the attending physician) and the learner (e.g., the resident physician). While the broader medical education literature is brimming with techniques and tips for giving feedback down the chain of command, there is little information available that addresses the unique challenge of giving feedback to superiors in the GME setting.

Giving Feedback to Superiors Within Business and Management Sectors

What does the leadership and management literature say about the importance of receiving honest, timely upward feedback?

It is interesting to note that within the business and management literature, accurate, honest upward feedback was found to be mostly absent. When it did occur, the feedback was usually inaccurately positive. Not only were senior managers unaware

---

S.S. Brody, D.O.
Department of Health Informatics, University of Miami
Miller School of Medicine, Plantation, FL, USA

J. Oppenheimer, M.D.
Department of Anesthesiology, University of Miami
Miller School of Medicine, Plantation, FL, USA

M.C. Lewis, M.D. (✉)
University of Florida, College of Medicine Jacksonville,
655 West 8th St Jacksonville, FL 32209, USA
e-mail: michael.lewis@jax.ufl.edu

of the distortions in the accuracy of the feedback, but they were unwilling to contemplate the possibility that the inconsistencies did indeed exist. Managers were found to have an exaggerated impression of how much upward feedback they received and were surprised to discover that they actually (intentionally or unintentionally) discouraged the transmission of corrective feedback [1].

Several negative consequences caused by a lack of upward feedback are identified in the business and management literature. One such consequence was "groupthink" described by Janis [2, 3]. Janis found that groups insulated from critical upward and outside feedback developed illusions of their own invulnerability, often distorting information to fit their rationalization for a certain behavior, and had excessive self-confidence in the quality of their decision-making. It follows that a group so inclined would also have a tendency to disparage and devalue, and ultimately not seek criticism from subordinates, since it would conflict with the group's ideal self-image and depart from its well-entrenched norms [1, 2].

Ingratiation theory has been cited as a barrier to upward feedback by Jones and Kassing. They proposed that those with a lower level of status habitually exaggerated the extent to which they agreed with the opinions and actions of higher status people as a means of acquiring influence with them. In particular, when subordinates contemplated giving corrective upward feedback, they considered whether or not it would result in retaliation or whether it would be perceived as constructive. This posed the question of whether trusting relationships existed within the hierarchy. The presence or absence of trust determined the availability and efficacy of upward feedback. Without trust, such communication was limited [4, 5].

Kluger and DeNisi provided evidence that upward feedback was most likely to result in performance improvements when it directed its attention to required behavioral changes rather than targeting a superior's personality or habits: [6] that is to say, when upward corrective feedback was directed at the behavior, not the person, it was more likely to prove effective.

How subordinates perceived giving feedback to superiors was considered in the work of Smith and Fortunato. Those subordinates who valued the process viewed upward feedback as a role appropriate activity, understood the process and content of upward feedback, and had ample opportunity to observe their supervisor. Moreover these individuals were more likely to believe in their ability to provide honest upward feedback and, as a result, were more inclined to do so [7].

Giving Feedback to Superiors Within Medical Education

Within the current medical education literature, there are very few articles directly addressed to the area of giving feedback to superiors. One such study was performed with first- and second-year medical students at the Virginia Commonwealth University. The researchers reported that students felt comfortable providing anonymous feedback to program faculty (e.g., a faculty lecturer), but fewer felt comfortable giving feedback to a preceptor with whom the student worked one-on-one.

Students commented that providing feedback to their preceptors was important but uncomfortable due to the lack of anonymity, which students said limited their candor on preceptorship evaluations [8].

Giving Feedback to Superiors Within Anesthesiology

Informal interviews with medical educators within anesthesiology reveal that the majority of educational interactions within an anesthesiology training program are one-on-one, team-based, and/or ongoing throughout the duration of GME training. Thus, giving corrective feedback to superiors in anesthesiology may be even more difficult than in other training programs.

The informal interviews revealed another unique facet of GME training within anesthesiology that complicates upward feedback: the emphasis on teaching technical skills. Much of the early training of anesthesiology residents involves mastery of a wide variety of technical skills. Teaching invasive procedures like central line placement may be standardized to ensure sterile technique and patient safety and may inherently involve less variability across attending anesthesiologists. However, when there is no single correct technique to complete a task, many different techniques may be taught within the training program. Commonplace tasks such as securing an endotracheal tube can have large inter-practitioner variability without any discernible difference in efficacy. While residents will inevitably be exposed to many techniques for "taping the tube," attending anesthesiologists may insist that this task be completed "their way." Even at the point where residents feel they have developed their own effective techniques, residents may still feel compelled to comply with the attending's preferences to avoid sending implicit upward feedback. Attending anesthesiologists who insist that tasks large and small be completed "their way" do not foster an environment conducive to upward feedback.

Due to the dependent relationship between teacher and learner and emphasis on teamwork in anesthesiology training programs, residents are reluctant to give feedback that could jeopardize them in the long term. It is less risky for residents to acquiesce to attending preferences than assert their own probably, equally valid preferences. However, it can be hypothesized that, when effective strategies for eliciting and soliciting feedback are used by anesthesiology attendings, this dependent relationship can be leveraged for the good of both the teacher and the learner.

Ongoing Research at University of Miami Miller School of Medicine on Giving Feedback to Superiors

The lack of information regarding giving feedback to superiors in the medical education literature led physicians and educators at the University of Miami Miller School of Medicine (UMMSM) to dig deeper to understand the barriers to giving

Table 11.1 Reasons medical educators cite for learners' reluctance to give upward feedback

1. Fear of retaliation, effect on evaluations or career
2. Lack of receptiveness of the teacher
3. Hurtfulness or threat of a message about teaching, clinical competence, or personal behavior
4. Skills of both teacher and learner in dealing with feedback
5. Our concept of feedback as one-way, corrective criticism instead of bidirectional and formative
6. Feedback is not part of a routine, scheduled interaction or conversation
7. Failure to understand the perspective of the other

feedback to superiors and how they can be overcome. To this end, medical educators worldwide were queried via the Dr-Ed Listserv to gather their impressions as to why learners were reluctant to give feedback to teachers. The main reasons expressed are listed in Table 11.1.

Armed with the insights gleaned from the Dr-Ed respondents, focus groups were organized with residents from six different residency programs at UMMSM. After analyzing the focus group data with NVivo software, three distinct themes emerged:

1. Barriers to giving feedback to superiors
2. Strategies teachers can use to solicit and elicit feedback from learners
3. Strategies learners can use to give feedback to teachers

Barriers to Giving Feedback to Superiors

Our study indicated that two significant barriers to giving feedback to superiors exist within medical education:

1. Relationship between the threat of the message and the receptivity of the recipient
2. Cultural aspects within the organization that do not support giving feedback to superiors

Barrier 1: Relationship Between the Threat of the Message and the Receptivity of the Recipient

Before conducting the resident focus groups, the researchers logically assumed that if the threat of the message content from the resident was low (e.g., "Rounds went a little long today."), and the attending was open to corrective feedback (e.g., an attending who had previously expressed interest in becoming a better educator), then it would *not* be difficult for the resident to give feedback to the attending. This describes the "Least Difficult" scenario seen in Fig. 11.1.

11 Giving Feedback to Superiors-Attending Evaluation

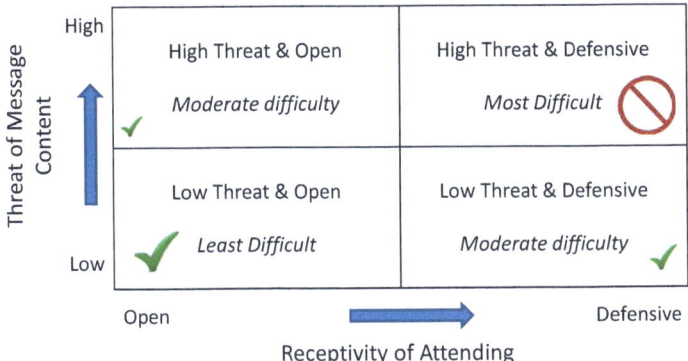

Fig. 11.1 Effect of message threat and defensiveness on giving *corrective* feedback to superiors

It was further hypothesized that as the threat of the message content from the resident increased, and the receptivity of the attending to corrective feedback decreased, then it would become ever more difficult for the resident to give corrective feedback to the attending.

The "Most Difficult" category was postulated to be the extreme, rare case when a resident would not give any feedback to the attending for fear of retaliation or similar unwanted repercussions (Fig. 11.1).

What was actually discovered through analysis of the preliminary data from resident focus groups was that residents did not feel comfortable giving feedback to an attending regardless of the threat of the message or the receptivity of the attending (Fig. 11.2).

Qualitative analysis of the preliminary data expanded the researchers' understanding of how residents defined "receptivity" to feedback:

- Age: younger attendings earlier in their careers where generally described as more open.
- Modernity of teaching style: residents described defensive attendings as "old school" and open attendings as "new school."
- Capability to synthesize and apply feedback: residents said they were more likely to give feedback to an attending who was considered to be capable of digesting and then applying corrective feedback.

The preliminary data also helped the researchers expand their understanding of the term "defensiveness" as it applied to attendings' receptivity to feedback

Residents consider a defensive attending to be:

- Retaliatory
- Prone to blame others for his/her mistakes
- Unable to synthesize feedback

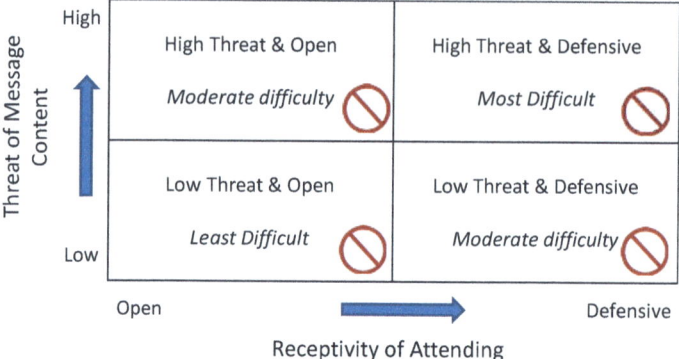

Fig. 11.2 Effect of message threat and defensiveness on giving *corrective* feedback to superiors

- Unable to apply feedback
- Prone to "shut down" the learner

Finally, the preliminary data also provided a deeper understanding of the "Threat of the Message." Residents believed that the most effective way to offer low threat, corrective feedback to an attending was by verbally praising desired behavior. The data showed that low threat messages were nearly always delivered using this technique, known as "positive reinforcement" [9]. In other words, residents tended to use verbal praise to increase the likelihood that a desired behavior will occur in the future under similar circumstances and did not feel that they could effectively provide verbal corrective feedback by any other method.

Examples of low threat messages included:

> It was important that you set expectations at the beginning of the rotation.
> I really appreciate you taking the time to show me how to do the physical exam.
> I really felt like I could contact you at any time with questions.

Naturally, the researchers believed that anonymous, written evaluations would be the residents' method of choice for providing corrective feedback to the attending. The data showed, however, that residents did not feel confident in the anonymity of such evaluations and almost never used them as a vehicle to provide corrective feedback. Even more so if the residency program or clinical team had few participants.

Barrier 2: Cultural Aspects Within the Organization That Do Not Support Giving Feedback to Superiors

Data from the preliminary focus groups with residents from six programs, including anesthesiology, at University of Miami indicated that the ability to give feedback to superiors was largely dependent upon the culture of the organization. A culture where a learner could give feedback to a superior would be defined by such characteristics as absence of the fear of reprisal or retaliation, the willingness of both teachers and learners to actively seek and give feedback as a stimulus for improvement, provision of protected time for feedback, and provision of a format (e.g., standardized form, script, or template) for teachers to solicit and elicit feedback from learners.

Willingness of faculty and residents to provide and receive feedback may also be influenced by an individual's own culture or ethnicity. In such instances, even practical changes to the institutional culture such as those listed above may fall short. Advanced, culturally competent and specific initiatives may be needed to overcome these types of barriers.

Strategies for Teachers to Solicit and Elicit Feedback from Learners

Analysis of the data from the resident focus groups not only identified the barriers to giving feedback to superiors but also revealed six specific strategies teachers can use to solicit and elicit feedback from their learners:

1. Ask about specific behaviors instead of global performance.
    Avoid asking general questions such as "So how am I doing?"
2. Ask learners to help you make a specific behavioral change.
    Choose a specific behavior or habit you'd like to fine-tune and ask learners to provide feedback:
    - I have a tendency to…so could you watch out for…
    - Please be on the lookout for…
    - Other learners have commented on my past evaluations that I…
3. Ask to "borrow good ideas" used by other teachers.
    Don't be afraid that you are "giving away power" by admitting that you can learn from other teachers and colleagues.
4. Emphasize professional responsibility to one another.
    Remember: today's learner is tomorrow's colleague.
5. Be welcoming of feedback.
    A teacher encourages feedback from learners when he or she receives the feedback gladly.
    Avoid defensiveness and excuses.
6. Establish pilot–copilot relationship [10].
    A plane must be flown by both a pilot *and* a copilot to avoid a crash.

    - Decrease the power distance between the teacher and learner by sharing thought processes and concerns with learners, and encouraging learners to do the same.
    - Consider and practice cultural competence: keep in mind that some learners come from cultures where giving feedback to a superior is forbidden, no matter how open the recipient appears to be.

Strategies for Residents to Use when Giving Feedback to a Superior

When the preliminary resident focus group data were correlated with information from informal interviews with medical educators, six strategies for learners to use when giving feedback to superiors consistently emerged.

1. Test the waters.
   Start by offering non-threatening feedback to gauge the attending's receptivity.
   One quote from a focus group participant was particularly pertinent:

   …when you do bring up [an] issue, if the attending doesn't take your opinion at all, doesn't consider your opinion at all…that's the end of the communication, that's the end of the line. I'm sort of powerless to bring up anything else. And I WON'T bring up anything else in the future, and then that affects patient care.

2. Be patient and wait for the right opportunity.
   Consider confidentiality and scheduling issues.
   Quote from focus group participant when mentioning the "Time Out" as a good opportunity in the operating room setting to offer upward feedback:

   It's definitely an opportunity to correct mistakes [that] come up. And I think that in my experience everyone in the OR is paying attention during that time…I've had mistakes corrected during the time out. I've corrected mistakes during a time out, conversely. In my opinion…it's a valuable exercise. It's something I take seriously. I think we all take [it] seriously in [our program].

3. Turn feedback into a question.
   For example, instead of saying, "Sit down rounds are not effective for me," rephrase as "I really learn well from bedside rounds. Could we try that tomorrow?"
   Quote from focus group participant who mentioned that by making reference to the current literature, a resident can avoid the appearance of exerting authority over the attending:

   …you're not just blindly questioning them, which I think can be construed to some [attendings] as insulting. And that way you're like, "Oh, well I saw this [in the literature]. What do you think about it?"…You're asking them their opinion about something else. [It's] like giving them another option.

4. Choose areas that are not sensitive for the attending.
   Avoid feedback that directly addresses the attending's personality or character traits.
   Quotes from focus group participants from two different residency programs:

   The feedback that I find easiest to give to attendings or more senior residents is … when they're actively involved in teaching. So, the example that I used is like when they are teaching a **technical skill**.

   I think it's easy to give feedback [about] **management of patients**…I'm not saying that every one of our attendings is perfectly open to feedback when it comes to discussion of medical care for the patient, but I think that…compared to other specialties, I think that our attendings value our feedback in that area.

5. Don't just state the problem, propose a solution.
   Quote from focus group participant:

   > Instead of going, 'This is not working. Let's try plan B.' I usually approach it from, 'Well this is interesting. We've tried Plan A. How about, in addition to that, trying B? Can we do a trial run of B?' Because then what you're communicating is, 'I appreciate what you've done. Can we try something more?' Instead of, 'Everything you've done up until now has not worked and it's a mess.'

6. A brief word of praise and gratitude can give a teacher the confidence and courage to try new techniques and strive to be better.
   Teachers have their doubts and fears just like residents do.

The Feedback Filter

The efficacy of every skill in teaching depends upon *the quality of the relationship* between teacher and learner. All feedback passes through a "relationship filter" as it makes its way to the recipient. This filter represents the quality of the relationship between the teacher and learner (Fig. 11.3). The residents in our focus groups mentioned that, when they have a good rapport with the attending, residents are much more likely to test the waters and give corrective/constructive feedback. Conversely, no matter the skills, strategies, or number of attempts to give feedback, if the quality of the relationship between the teacher and learner is poor, the feedback may be interpreted negatively by the recipient.

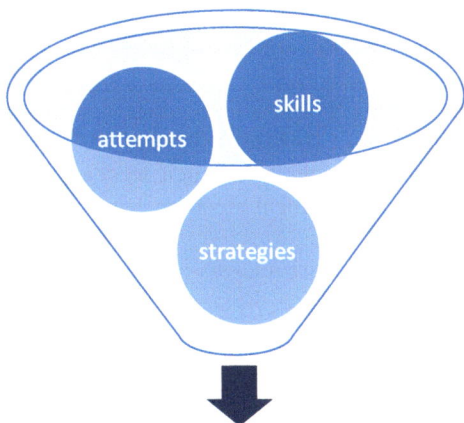

Fig. 11.3 Feedback filter

Residents from focus groups across many departments mentioned that it is easiest to give corrective upward feedback to attendings with whom they had friendly and respectful, but less deferential, professional relationships. Inevitably there are some teachers who feel that it is not the learner's role to help the teacher improve his or her teaching or clinical skills. These teachers will not receive corrective upward feedback. However, when learners identify this high power distance separating them from the teacher, corrective feedback, no matter how well crafted and strategized, will go unspoken.

Giving, Soliciting, and Eliciting Feedback Are Skills

Much like placement of a central line or intubation, giving and receiving feedback is a skill that must be learned and mastered through deliberate practice [11]. Deliberate practice involves three steps:

a. Practice at the appropriate level
b. Performance assessment that is immediate and informative
c. Opportunities for repetition and correction of errors

Physicians can improve their skills of giving, soliciting, and eliciting feedback within anesthesiology training programs by creating opportunities for deliberate practice. These focused efforts will not only improve the quality of the individual attending's teaching skill but also create a more positive and productive environment for the program as a whole.

Conclusion

Clearly for anesthesiology residents, like all subordinates, giving corrective feedback to superiors is a difficult task. Likewise, it is both challenging and sometimes uncomfortable for attendings to solicit and elicit feedback from trainees. At the same time, the business and management literature demonstrates the imperative for upward feedback.

Currently, there is scant literature addressing this issue as it relates to GME. Our research at the UMMSM illustrates the significant challenges our residents face when offering corrective feedback up the hierarchy. These barriers come from both the learners' concern for repercussions and teachers' unwillingness or disinterest in receiving feedback from learners. Structural and cultural barriers are especially acute in anesthesiology training programs. The combination of daily one-on-one interactions, emphasis on operating room efficiency, and team-based care over years of training may hamper trainees' motivation to provide upward feedback.

The next step in this line of investigation is to create and implement an intervention based on the strategies for soliciting and eliciting upward feedback. A cultural shift within a department or an institution may increase the likelihood of feedback given and received. Investment by faculty in the value of upward feedback, a global expectation that upward feedback must be given by learners, and frequent protected time dedicated to giving and receiving feedback are essential to the success and enrichment of anesthesiology training programs.

References

1. Tourish D, Robson P. Critical upward feedback in organisations: processes, problems and implications for communication management. J Comm Manag. 2004;8(2):150–67.
2. Aldag RJ, Fuller SR. Groupthink. Encyclopedia of applied psychology. New York: Elsevier; 2004. p. 143–51.
3. Mackin D. The team building tool kit: tips and tactics for effective workplace teams. New York: AMACOM; 2007.
4. Jones EE, Baumeister RF. The self-monitor looks at the ingratiator. J Pers. 1976;44:654–74.
5. Kassing J. From the look of things: assessing perceptions of organizational dissenters. Manag Comm Q. 2001;14:442–70.
6. Kluger AN, DeNisi A. The effects of feedback interventions upon performance: a historical review, a meta-analysis, and a preliminary feedback intervention theory. Psychol Bull. 1996;119:254–84.
7. Smith AFR, Fortunato V. Factors influencing employee intentions to provide honest upward feedback ratings. J Bus Psychol. 2008;22:191–207.
8. Willett RM, Lawson SR, Gary JS, Kancitis IA. Medical student evaluation of faculty in student-preceptor pairs. Acad Med. 2007;82(10 Suppl):S30–3.
9. Skinner BF. Two types of conditioned reflex: a reply to Konorski and Miller. J Gen Psychol. 1937;16:272–9.
10. Gladwell M. Outliers: the story of success. New York: Little, Brown and Company; 2008. p. 177–274.
11. Ericsson KA, Krampe RT, Tesch-Römer C. The role of deliberate practice in the acquisition of *expert* performance. Psychol Rev. 1993;100:363–406.

Chapter 12
The Place for Simulation Teaching

Judy G. Johnson

> I hear and I forget. I see and I remember. I do and I understand—Confucius

Introduction

The proliferation of social media and technology has changed the way educators teach, how students learn, and the way teachers and students communicate. Traditional methods, i.e., long days sitting in the classroom, feet under desk, squarely planted due north at the chalk board, teachers billowing words of knowledge on complex issues, have been replaced. Technology has provided a plethora of high fidelity sights and sounds, changing the face of education. Tablet computers with their fast processors, internet connectivity, and large touch-screen displays can function as powerful graphing calculators, video players, and photo editors [1]. Thousands of college lectures, videos, and textbooks are available as electronic textbooks, replacing the standard hard covers. Educational curricula that combine standard textbooks with interactive content are expanding. Along with this technologic surge, simulation has evolved to the forefront of education. This widespread growth has paved the way for differing industries, involving various venues, to become immersed in simulation. Most simulations are computer based [2] and often involve multistage algorithms that calculate performance based on the decisions of the participants [3]. With integration of simulation training into an existing course curriculum, educators are finding bold and innovative alternatives to the learning experience.

J.G. Johnson, M.D. (✉)
Department of Anesthesiology, School of Medicine, Louisiana State University Health Sciences Center, 1542 Tulane Avenue, Suite 659, New Orleans, LA 70112, USA
e-mail: jjohn1@lsuhsc.edu

Simulation

Simulation has been defined as the imitative representation of the functioning of one system or process by means of the functioning of another; a computer simulation of an industrial process [4]. Simulation enables participants to learn through interactive experiences (Fig. 12.1). This virtual medium promotes various types of skills to be learned and exercised in a non-threatening way. With differing industries and various objectives to be achieved, it is hard to outline a specific skill-set that will address all goals. However, the business industry stands behind four key areas that participants must strive to obtain in order for the simulation program to be a success: [5] (1) *business awareness*, e.g., the process of having some control and decision-making ability in a virtual reality setting; (2) *time management and organization*, thus, sessions are timed, which will test the participant's skill in submitting decisions within an allotted time frame; (3) *problem solving*, where simulation will often present crafty scenarios that must be thought through logically with successful resolution, and (4) *team coordination*, e.g., the ability to work as a team or group; whereby application of communication skills and delegation of tasks for purpose-directed problem solving are foremost.

Most educators understand the important role experience plays in the learning process. David Kolb, an educational theorist, helped define the idea of "experiential education." Learning is aimed at the development of problem solving through active participation, prior exposure, and knowledge. There are components of intellect and emotion when learning from past experience. Individuals are encouraged to directly involve themselves in the experience and then to reflect on it [6]. Simulation provides this educational opportunity.

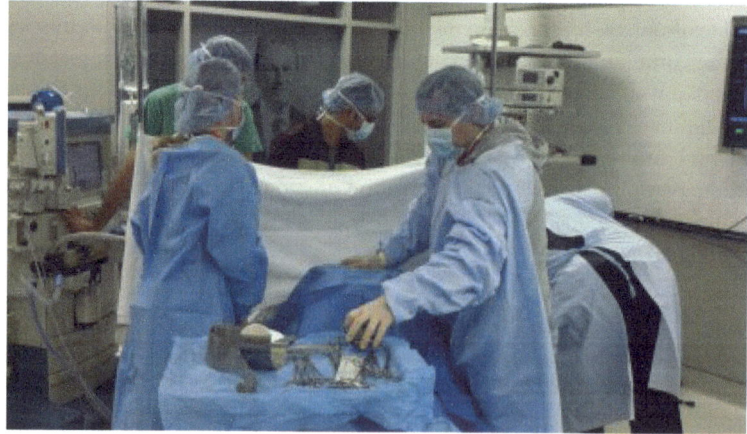

Fig. 12.1 LSU Anesthesiology residents participate in an obstetric simulation case

Simulation-Based Medical Education

As medical technologies expand, demands on medical educators are changing and the performance of the healthcare profession is being redefined. Contributing factors for this change include: changes in healthcare delivery and academic environments that limit patient availability for educational opportunities; attention focused on the problem of medical errors and the need to improve patient safety; and the paradigm shift to outcomes-based education with its requirements for assessment and demonstration of competence [7]. Simulation centers for training have become part of the medical education fabric.

Scalese et al. describe medical simulation as an aim to imitate real patients, anatomic regions, or clinical tasks, and/or to mirror the real-live circumstances in which medical services are rendered [7]. A wide variety of medical conditions and ailments can be obtained on demand; no more waiting for the real patients with specific conditions to venture to the hospital. *Simulators do not become tired or embarrassed or behave unpredictably as might real, especially ill, patients, and therefore they provide a standardized experience for all* [8].

Integration of Training Simulation

Traditionally, medical schools have provided a passive educational experience, focusing more on academics than on hands-on clinical training, especially in the first 2 years. However, integration of training simulations has provided many benefits; giving a new fresh perspective, as well as being entertaining, and exciting [9], to being readily available at any time and reproducing a wide variety of clinical conditions (Fig. 12.2) [7].

Whether these programmed simulations fall under the category of profoundly simple to astutely complex, a structural format of the training session is warranted. Such a structure may be:

Introduction: The director gives an introduction which comprises of meeting the participants, defining goals and objectives, and relaying the purpose behind the training.
Simulation case: The envelopment of participation, comprising a realistic environment with the acquisition of skills being practiced and knowledge being tested.
Reflection: A summary of events, a time of retrospective contemplation and evaluation of individual and collaborative skills, in an atmosphere conducive to learning.

Curriculum Design

Sheila Chauvin, Ph.D., Director and Professor of the Office of Medical Education Research Development at Louisiana State University Health Sciences Center, holds a Statewide Simulation Faculty Development Program which provides insight

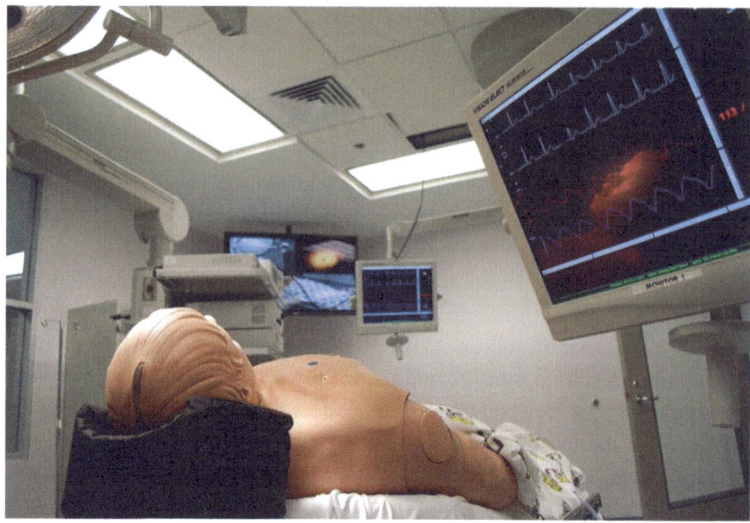

Fig. 12.2 The Center for Advanced Practice at Louisiana State University Health Sciences Center in New Orleans, Louisiana is a source for integrated learning of medical students and residents at every stage of training

and guidance. She states, "that when faced with developing a curriculum design it is best to possibly start with the *End* in mind. In other words, what are the gaps that need to be filled? What goal must be accomplished?" [10] She relies on the widely adopted principles of educational and instructional design that is often represented in the ADDIE model [11]. The following five key elements help provide a systematic and practical approach that can be used effectively for developing and refining simulation-based training:

*A*ssess and analyze: This targets issues specific to the learners, the resources available, and the feasibility and receptivity to innovation and change. Obtaining this information may be through direct observation, surveys and interviews, program accreditation standards, and prior performance.

*D*esign: Design may be structured as follows:

1. Define the educational *context* in which the curriculum or course will be implemented.
2. Identify the *goals* to be addressed.
3. Develop specific, learner-centered and observable *objectives* that fit with the curriculum goals. Formulate SMART goals and objectives (i.e., Specific, Measurable, Achievable/Action-oriented, Relevant/Realistic, and Timely/Time-bound).

The process of developing goals and objectives will help to identify the learning context that will be best for achieving the intended education and training outcomes. Development of an *assessment* framework can be challenging. Direct observation-based performance, endorsed standard setting, collection of example behaviors, and acquisition of factual knowledge by testing are all reliable tools. Revisiting various aspects of the assessment tools to guarantee appropriate evidence of validity and reliability is essential [12].

*D*evelop: Defining the core content to be addressed and the *methods* of delivery help in the development process. For example the content can be competencies, best practices and/or any prerequisite experiences, knowledge, or skills required for success. Resources and materials are vitally important in simulation. In order to engage the learner in a realistic environment, equipment and various props, actors and clinical supplies may be needed. *The high fidelity stationary simulators such as the METI Human Patient Simulators, have the advantage of providing a more realistic environment without the challenge of transporting equipment and materials, or finding additional space in the hospital setting. Simulation sessions can be easily scheduled without interruption of demanding operating room availability* [13].

*I*mplement and deliver: Conducting a trial-run is beneficial and allows for refinement and adjustments to various aspects of the simulation scenario. Often the participants have input and helpful suggestions regarding the structural format, especially the introduction and reflection periods.

*E*valuate: This phase has both formative and summative assessments. These types of assessments lead to collaborative feedback among faculty and learners. Through utilization of assessment tools and collation of data, both learner performance and program effectiveness can be evaluated.

Dr. Chauvin points out that the ADDIE model is cyclical in nature and to achieve desired enhancement and/or expansion, the process can be repeated and refined [10].

Clinical Skills

Medical education covers a broad spectrum of concepts and skills, involving not only academic and scientific training but also the acquisition of clinical skills related directly to patient care. Constraints on medical education such as limited duty-hours, reduced patient volumes, or variable acuity and complexity of illness may produce gaps in resident medical knowledge and skills. The historical acceptance of practicing various invasive procedures and techniques on "real patients" has been altered with the help of simulation-based medical education (SBME) allowing the inexperienced student to master their skills in a risk-free atmosphere.

Recent meta-analyses suggested that clinical training alone is inferior to clinical training plus SBME. McGaghie et al. concluded SBME with deliberate practice is superior to traditional clinical medical education in achieving specific clinical skill acquisition goals [14]. "Deliberate practice is shooting for expertise; it's not so much quantity but quality" [10]. Attributes of deliberate practice are defined by McGaghie et al., as highly motivated learners, with well-defined objectives at appropriate levels of difficulty. There must be a focused practice with focused feedback that includes measurable educational standards. Feedback contributions from the trainee and trainer, self-reflection, correction, and repetition are essential elements. *The goal of deliberate practice in a CME mastery-learning context is to require constant improvement of skill and knowledge rather than maintenance of a minimal level* [15].

SBME has been an effective method to boost clinical skills [16]. As development and dissemination of educational programs involving simulation for clinical skills continues to evolve, the expectation is that it will improve medical training, patient safety, and quality of care. Singer et al. compared the bedside critical care competency of first-year internal medicine residents who completed a simulation-based intervention to traditionally trained third-year residents who completed training alone. Their findings demonstrated a higher clinical competency in the first-year residents who underwent simulation training. These results suggest that bedside competency is not solely a function of training time and lecture attendance [17].

Team Approach in Simulated Learning

SBME often draws upon a team-oriented approach. The acceptance of simulated learning and the recognition of different team-oriented roles in modern healthcare have converged in the form of simulation-based team training (SBTT) [18]. Teamwork consists of individual members' interrelated thoughts, actions, and feelings allowing them to function as a coordinated group with adaptive performance that leads to value-added outcomes. Five key features of teamwork have been called the "Big Five": (1) Leadership, (2) Performance monitoring, (3) Backup behavior, (4) Adaptability, and (5) Orientation. Furthermore, "shared mental models, "closed loop" communication, and mutual trust support the coordination of these team processes" [16–18].

Salas et al. designate eight evidence-based principles for team training. These principles include: (1) Focus training content on critical teamwork competences, (2) Emphasize teamwork and team processes over task work, (3) Guide training based on desired team-based learning outcomes and organizational resources, (4) Incorporate hands-on, guided practice, (5) Match similar on-the-job mental processes and simulation-based training content to augment training relevance and transfer to practice, (6) Provide both outcome- and behavior-based feedback, (7) Evaluate training impact through clinical outcomes and work behaviors, (8) Reinforce desired teamwork behaviors through coaching and performance evaluation [18–20].

Participants

Multiple studies have demonstrated a high satisfaction level among the participants involved in educational experiences through simulation. As Butler, et al. [21], describe, "*It is important to note that "beating the game" should not be a primary aim for anyone taking part in a simulation; the focus should be directed toward everyone gaining some useful and relevant knowledge that they can take away and use in their daily lives*." Both Hynes [22] and Neal [23] relay that competitive elements help motivate and inspire the student. A bit of "rivalry" between teams or individuals improves the learning and adds an ingredient of drama and fun.

Making participants active and responsible for their own learning while ensuring they address important issues and extract maximum learning during debriefing is essential. Data from surveys of participants indicate that perceived skills of the debriefer have the highest independent correlation to the perceived overall quality of the simulation experience [24].

Facilitator

This role of "facilitator" is essential to the learning process and lends credibility to the simulation experience. Fanning et al. describe how facilitators aim to guide and direct rather than to lecture. "Unlike the traditional classroom teacher, facilitators tend to position themselves not as authorities or experts, but rather as co-learners. This more fraternal approach may be most productive where the learning objective is behavioural change" [24]. Studies from Fanning contend that formal courses and refresher courses in facilitation are probably universally warranted. "In addition to the formal education of facilitators, techniques such as the pairing of an expert with novice facilitators, early in their career, to give guidance and direction, are important" [24].

Generic factors influence the work of the facilitator in the debriefing process. These factors include, but may not be limited to: "the objective of the experiential exercise, the complexity of the scenarios, the experience level of the participants as individuals or a team, the familiarity of the participants with the simulation environment, time available for the session, the role of simulations in the overall curriculum, individual personalities and relationships, if any between/among the participants [25]."

Debriefing

The post-simulation discussion is based on the concept of reflection on an event or activity and subsequent analysis. Debriefing is widely accepted as the most essential component in simulation training and is the foundation for experiential learning [26]. Debriefing facilitates participants' ability to relate their training experiences to daily practice [24]. An after-action debriefing format is described by Paige et al. [25] as consisting of three components: the introduction, the discussion, and closure. The discussion component was additionally compartmentalized into four phases:

1. *Engagement*: immediately engage the entire team.
2. *Focus*: identification of specific teamwork competencies.
3. *Reflection and critique*: reflect on various teamwork competencies and how to enhance effectiveness.
4. *Application*: commitment to apply knowledge and skills to everyday practice.

The debriefing instructor requires both structure and specific techniques to optimize learning during this time of reflection. Raemer et al. state the "debriefing by competent instructors is considered important to maximize the learning opportunities arising from simulated events." [27] Dieckmann et al. [28] report the considerable variation between the perceived ideal role of the debriefer and what is actually executed during real debriefing sessions exist. They go on to predict that "as simulation becomes more widely used in healthcare as a means of both formative and summative assessment, a reliable and valid way to assess the efficacy and quality of the debriefing becomes more important". The timing of the debriefing sessions has varied in their approach. Van Heukelom et al. found that students felt that the debriefing session was more effective and beneficial after the simulation session was complete as opposed to interruptions during the session. In-simulation debriefing led to an alteration of the "realism" of the simulation [29].

In the endeavor to develop common guidelines, researchers at Harvard developed the widely known debriefing assessment tool entitled "Debriefing Assessment for Simulation in Healthcare" (DASH). This tool includes six debriefing elements crucial to facilitation of an effective debriefing session. Early research has shown that this tool has strong interrator reliability and preliminary evidence of validity [30]. The DASH tracks and rates key elements of a debriefing. These include whether and how the instructor:

1. Establishes an engaging learning environment
2. Maintains an engaging learning environment
3. Structures debriefing in an organized way
4. Provokes engaging discussions
5. Identifies and explores performance gaps
6. Helps trainees achieve or sustain good future performance

DASH Handbook and Rating Forms can be found on the Harvard simulation website [31].

Online debriefing tutorials can also be found. For example, the American Heart Association course focuses on "a learner-centered debriefing model, draws on evidence-based findings from behavioral science, focuses on critical thinking and encourages participants to analyze their performance and motivations. Structured and Supported Debriefing teaches advanced life support instructors how to facilitate an effective debriefing of their students within 10 minutes after a skills practice session" [32].

Application of Simulation

Training simulations have been used in a wide variety of high risk performance industries such as aviation, military units, business, driving instruction, and nuclear power plants. The ability to incorporate simulation technology into training and assessment programs not only enhances the individual's skills but also promotes an environment of collaborative teamwork [33–35].

A growing body of evidence shows that clinical skills acquired in simulation settings transfer directly to improved patient care practices and better patient outcomes [36].

Ultimately, the goals of SBME are defined in terms of enhancing patient safety, improving medical care, and boosting physician performance. The assumption is that learning from mistakes in a simulated environment will reduce occurrences of errors in real life and will provide learners with the correct attitude and skills to cope competently with those mistakes that cannot be prevented.

The paradigm shift toward outcomes-based education throughout healthcare has prompted academic institutions and hospital credentialing committees to delineate benchmark indicators of competency. Addressing accountability of physicians [37], specialty boards are placing emphasis on simulation modalities for evaluation of competency and the ability to obtain and continue certification.

Certification

The American Society of Anesthesiology (ASA) has embraced SBME with the advent of Maintenance of Certification in Anesthesiology. A website on Simulation Education is devoted to this endeavor.

The American Society of Anesthesiologists' Simulation Education Program is the culmination of consultation among leaders in anesthesia simulation. The Program advocates the promotion of learning through simulation and specifically approves programs of quality in anesthesiology simulation training. The Committee on Simulation Education oversees the Simulation Education Network that provides training to satisfy the American Board of Anesthesiology's Maintenance of Certification in Anesthesiology (MOCA®) requirements [38].

One component of this re-certification is to be an active participant of the simulation experience. These simulation sessions are held at designated and approved training sites around the country. Performance during these simulation sessions is only one component to certification. The physician must take the acquisition of skills and knowledge learned in SBME and implement change in their daily practice.

The ASA has endorsed simulation centers located throughout the United States that offer courses that help to fulfill one requirement of the American Board of Anesthesiology's (ABA) Maintenance of Certification in Anesthesiology Program (MOCA®) Part IV. The endorsement process by the ASA Committee for Simulation Education is extensive and covers the center's mission, educational offerings, curriculum development, instructor and course effectiveness, program leadership, and infrastructure. Members of ASA and the simulation community will benefit from this Program as it promotes patient safety through refinement of training and team enhancement [38].

Anesthesiology is not the only specialty focusing on simulation for certification. The American Board of Internal Medicine (ABIM) is incorporating medical simulation technology for Interventional Cardiologist to evaluate competence.

ABIM has introduced an exciting new option for interventional cardiology diplomates to earn credit toward completion of the Self-Evaluation of Medical Knowledge requirement for Maintenance of Certification. Interventional Cardiology Simulations is the first-ever ABIM-developed lab-based simulation that provides an opportunity to perform cases that mirror what an interventional cardiologist would typically face in daily practice. This is the first time ABIM is using simulation to evaluate physician competence.

Medical Simulation Corporation's SimSuite® technology replicates a real-life catheterization lab suite, and the five case scenarios developed by ABIM include common problems faced by interventional cardiologists. Physicians complete the Interventional Cardiology Simulations onsite at one of Medical Simulation Corporation's six SimSuite® education centers or at several cardiology meetings and conferences throughout the year [39].

The Department of Medicine at the University of British Columbia reported on the development and implementation of physical examination stations that combine simulation technology in the form of digitized cardiac auscultation videos with a standardized patient assessment for the 2003 Royal College of Physicians and Surgeons of Canada's Comprehensive Objective Examination in Internal Medicine. "The candidates' mean scores for both types of stations were similar, as were the mean discrimination indices for both types of stations, suggesting that the combined stations were of a testing standard similar to the traditional stations. Combining examinations on standardized patients with simulation technology may be one approach to the assessment of clinical competence in high-stakes testing situations" [40].

At the Louisiana State Health Sciences Center, Paige and his team have been active in running multidisciplinary simulation-based operating room team training. Team coordination, cohesive functioning, and nontechnical skills are some of the focused training strategies. Nontechnical skills are the combination of those cognitive and interpersonal skills that complement each team member's technical skills to contribute to a safe effective operative intervention. They form the foundation on which team interaction and dynamics are built. Nontechnical skills are not innately derived; instead, they can be acquired through teaching and training, much like technical skills are learned. Paige concludes that within today's complex, dynamic systems of healthcare, physicians must draw on more than their technical skills to succeed. Instead, they must bring key nontechnical skills to bear to promote team-based competencies within the OR team. This multi-professional nature of practice allows each profession to improve team-based attitudes among participants as well as team-based behaviors within the actual operating room environment [41].

Considerations and Outcomes-Based Education

During simulation sessions, many components are to be considered such as judgment under pressure, medical decision-making, situational awareness, teamwork, and professional behavior. Tichy and Bennis, in their book entitled "Judgment,

How Winning Leaders Make Great Calls," describe judgment as being a three dimensional process: *time, domain and constituencies*. They state *time* requires preparation, the decision, and the execution. Three *domains*, which the leader must confront after the decision is made, is judgments about people, judgments about strategy and judgments about crisis. Finally, the third dimension consists of *constituencies*. A leader must interact with differing constituencies, consider their various interests, and manage those relationships to make successful judgment calls [42].

A framework to improve the ability to make judgments relies on four types of knowledge: [42]

1. Self-knowledge: personal values and goals
2. Social network knowledge: regarding those who surround the decision maker
3. Organizational knowledge: knowledge about people at all levels
4. Contextual knowledge: knowledge about other stakeholders.

Conceptually, these elements of leadership, judgment calls, and team coordination all interplay and should declare themselves during a simulated environment.

SBME Research Groups are emerging in many medical specialties, including anesthesiology, emergency medicine, internal medicine, obstetrics and gynecology, pediatrics and surgery. Research programs produce most valuable results when studies are thematic, sustained, and cumulative [43]. These efforts are on-going. One important question that Scalese et al. highlight in their article is the "predictive validity" of simulation. *Will performance on a given assessment predict future performance in actual practice?* [7] The authors point to two studies using virtual reality (VR) surgical simulation with showed significant improvement in performance which translated to improved operating room performance among the participants [44, 45].

Recently Mcgaghie et al. [36], through qualitative synthesis of SBME translational science research which employs a critical review approach to literature aggregation, concluded simulation improved patient safety and provided better patient care. He highlights many studies from 2000 to 2010 which utilize SBME and compared favorable patient outcomes. The report goes on to add that selection bias can contribute to confirmation bias, and that one must "be mindful about blind spots that can distort consensus conference proceedings and their conclusions".

Simulation-based interdisciplinary teams offer many advantages; it engages learners in lifelike experiences with varying fidelity designed to mimic real clinical encounters. McGaghie et al. suggest the need to enhance simulation-based medical education with deliberate practice. Deliberate practice embodies strong and consistent educational interventions grounded in information processing and behavioral theories of skill acquisition and maintenance [14].

Summary

Simulation; a copy of reality, but not really.

As medical education changes, so does the framework within the way the learners perceive and implement knowledge gained. SBME and team training has engaged the learner to develop group identity and collective cognitive processes. Ever-advancing technologies have provided tools for assessment of clinical skills, and enhancement of teaching practice. Educators have realized the scope of creativity and value in the use of these various tools. A high level of satisfaction among the participants and their teachers has been gained through simulation. The customary reliance on real patients for procedure oriented experience and the old adage approach of "see one, do one" has been challenged [7].

Are there drawbacks? Realization that the fidelity of a simulation is never completely identical to "the real thing" is due to engineering limitations, psychometric requirements, cost and time constraints [7]. McGaghie et al. stated it best, "Informed and effective use of SBME technology requires knowledge of best practices, perseverance, and attention to the values and priorities at play in one's local setting" [43].

Lastly, the ethical imperative must be acknowledged. Ziv et al. [46], in their review state balancing the needs of medical education and training with the obligation of providing optimal treatment and assurance of patient safety produces a fundamental ethical tension. *The use of simulation wherever feasible conveys a critical educational and ethical message to all: patients are to be protected whenever possible and they are not commodities to be used as conveniences of training.*

What great promise is on the horizon in the realm of simulation; enhancement of physician training, acquisition of clinical skills in a low-risk setting, improved patient safety, and the potential for better healthcare can be achieved.

References

1. Koleber J. More high schools implement iPad programs. usnews.com. 2011. http://www.usnews.com/education/blogs/high-school-notes/2011/09/07/more-high-schools-implement-ipad-programs. Accessed 7 Mar 2013.
2. Stuart JM. Business simulations—do they have a place in training? ezinearticles.com. 2007. http://ezinearticles.com/?Business-Simulations---Do-They-Have-A-Place-In-Training?&id=603769. Accessed 14 Mar 2013.
3. Fripp J. A future for business simulations? J Eur Ind Train. 1997;21(4):138–42.
4. Simulation. In: Merriam-Webster online. http://www.merriam-webster.com. Accessed 10 Mar 2013.
5. Heinz HJ. Business simulation means better senior managers at Heinz. J Eur Ind Train. 1999;23(1):46–7.
6. Loo R. A meta-analytic examination of Kolb's learning style preferences among business majors. J Educ Bus. 2002;77(5):252–6.
7. Scalese R, Obeso VT, Issenberg SB. Simulation technology for skills training and competency assessment in medical education. J Gen Intern Med. 2008;23 Suppl 1:46–9.
8. Collins JP, Harden RM. AMEE medical education guide no. 13: real patients, simulated patients and simulators in clinical examinations. Med Teach. 1998;20:508–21.
9. Wenzler I. Development of an asset management strategy for a network utility company: lessons from a dynamic business simulation approach. Simulat Gaming. 2005;36(1):75–90.

10. Chauvin S. Louisiana Statewide Simulation Faculty Development Program, Sponsored by the Simulation Medical Training and Education Council of LA, LSUHSC, New Orleans, LA, March 2012 (personal communication, 27 Feb 2013).
11. Kraiger K. Creating, implementing, and managing effective training and development systems in organizations: state-of-the-art lessons for practice. San Francisco: Jossey-Bass; 2002. p. 331–75.
12. Chauvin S. Assessment in simulation. In: Robertson HJ, Paige JT, Bok LR, editors. Simulation in radiology. New York: Oxford Press; 2012. p. 66–79.
13. Kozmenko V, Johnson J, Wyche M. High fidelity simulation as an effective tool in OR Leadership, Operating Room Leadership and Management. In: Kaye AD, Fox C, Urman R, editors. Operating Room Leadership and Management. New York, NY: Cambridge University Press; 2012. p. 274–8.
14. McGaghie WC, Issenberg SB, Cohen ER, Barsuk JH, Wayne DB. Does simulation-based medical education with deliberate practice yield better results than traditional clinical education? A meta-analytic comparative review of the evidence. Acad Med. 2011;86:706–11.
15. McGaghie W, Siddall MA, Mazmanian PE, Myers J. Lessons for continuing medical education from simulation research in undergraduate and graduate medical education: effectiveness of continuing medical education: American College of Chest Physicians evidence-based educational guidelines. Chest. 2009;135:62S–8.
16. Cook DA, Hatala R, Brydges R, et al. Technology-enhanced simulation for health professions education: a systematic review and meta-analysis. JAMA. 2011;306:978–88.
17. Singer BD, Corbridge TC, Schroedl CJ, Wilcox JE, Cohen ER, McGaghie WC, Wayne DB. First-year residents outperform third-year residents after simulation-based education in critical care medicine. Simul Healthc. 2013;8(2):67–71.
18. Eppich W, Howard V, Vozenilek J, Curran I. Simulation-based team training in healthcare. Simul Healthc. 2011;6 Suppl:S14–9.
19. Salas E, Wilson KA, Burke CA, Priest HA. Using simulation-based training to improve patient safety: what does it take? Jt Comm J Qual Patient Saf. 2005;31(7):363–71.
20. Salas E, Wilson KA, Lazzara EH, King HB, Augenstein JD, Robinson DW, et al. Simulation-based training for patient safety: 10 principles that matter. J Patient Saf. 2008;8(4):3–8.
21. Butler MJ, Reddy P. Developing critical understanding in JRM students: using innovative teaching methods to encourage deep approaches to study. J Eur Ind Train. 2010;34(8/9):772–89.
22. Hynes B, Costin Y, Birdthistle N. Practice-based learning in entrepreneurship education: a means of connecting knowledge producers and users. High Educ Skills Work base Learn. 2011;1(1):16–28.
23. Neal DJ. Group competitiveness and cohesion in a business simulation. Simulat Gaming. 1997;28(4):460–76.
24. Fanning RM, Gaba DM. The role of debriefing in simulation-based learning. Simul Healthc. 2007;2:115–25.
25. Gururaja RP, Yang T, Paige J, Chauvin S. Examining the effectiveness of debriefing at the point of care in simulation-based operating room team training. Agency of Research Healthcare and Quality. 2007. p. 1–18. www.ahrq.gov/…/resources/advances-in-patient-safety-2/vol3/TableofContents_Vol3.pdf - 11k _7.pdf. Accessed 5 Mar 2013.
26. Rall M, Manser T, Howard S. Key elements of debriefing for simulator training. Eur J Anesthesiol. 2000;17:516–7.
27. Raemer D, Anderson M, Cheng A, Fanning R, Nadkarni V, Savoldelli G. Research regarding debriefing as part of the learning process. Simul Healthc. 2011;6 Suppl:S52–7.
28. Dieckmann P, Molin FS, Lippert A, Ostergassrd D. Research regarding debriefing as part of the learning process. Med Teach. 2009;31(7):e287–94.
29. Van Heukelom JN, Begaz T, Treat R. Comparison of postsimulation debriefing versus in-simulation debriefing in medical simulation. Simul Healthc. 2010;5(2):91–7.
30. Brett-Fleegler M, Rudolph J, Eppich W, Monuteaux M, Fleegler E, Cheng A, Simon R. Debriefing assessment for simulation in healthcare: development and psychometric properties. Simul Healthc. 2012;7(5):288–94.

31. Harvard Center for Medical Simulation. Debriefing assessment for simulation in healthcare (DASH). http://www.harvardmedsim.org/debriefing-assesment-simulation-healthcare.php. Accessed 10 Mar 2013.
32. AHA. Structured and supported debriefing course. American Heart Association. http://www.heart.org/HEARTORG/CPRAndECC/InstructorNetwork/InstructorResources/Structured-and-Supported-Debriefing-Course_UCM_304285_Article.jsp. Accessed 6 Mar 2013.
33. Issenberg SB, McGaghie W, Hart MB, Mayer JW, Feiner JM, et al. Simulation technology for health care professional skills training and assessment. JAMA. 1999;282(9):861–6.
34. Ressler EK, Armstrong JE, Forsythe GB. Military mission rehearsal. In: Scalese RJ, Obeso V, Issenberg S. Simulation technology for skills training and competency assessment in medical education. J Gen Intern Med. 2008;23(Suppl 1):46–49.
35. Wachtel J. The future of nuclear power plant simulation in the United States. In: Walton DG, editor. Simulation for nuclear reactor technology. Cambridge: Cambridge University Press; 1985. p. 339–49.
36. McGaghie WC, Draycott TJ, Cunn WF, Lopex CM, Stefanidis D. Evaluating the impact of simulation on translational patient outcomes. Simul Healthc. 2011;6 Suppl:S42–7.
37. Scalese RJ, Issenberg SB. Effective use of simulations for the teaching and acquisition of veterinary professional and clinical skills. J Vet Med Educ. 2005;32(4):461–7.
38. ASA. Simulation education. ASA Education Center. American Society of Anesthesiology. http://education.asahq.org/simulation-education. Accessed 4 Mar 2013.
39. American Board of Internal Medicine. ABIM to use medical simulation technology to evaluate physician competence. American Board of Internal Medicine. http://www.abim.org/news/medical-simulation-technology-evaluate-physician-competence.aspx. Accessed 11 Mar 2013.
40. Hatala R, Kassen BO, Nishikawa J, Cole G, Issenberg SB. Incorporating simulation technology in a Canadian internal medicine specialty examination: a descriptive report. Acad Med. 2005;80(6):554–6.
41. Paige JT. Surgical team training: promoting high reliability with nontechnical skills. Surg Clin North Am. 2010;90(3):569–81.
42. Tichy N, Bennis W. Judgment, how winning leaders make great calls. New York, NY: Penguin Group Inc.; 2007. p. 1–40.
43. McGaghie WC, Issenberg SB, Petrusa ER, Scalese RJ. A critical review of simulation-based medical education research: 2003–2009. Med Educ. 2010;44(1):50–63.
44. Seymour NE, Gallagher AG, Roman SA, et al. Virtual reality training improves operating room performance: results of a randomized, double-blinded study. Ann Surg. 2002;236(4):458–64.
45. Grantcharov TP, Kristiansen VB, Bendix J, Bardram L, Rosenberg J. Randomized clinical trial of virtual reality simulation for laparoscopic skills training. Br J Surg. 2004;91(2):146–50.
46. Ziv A, Wolpe PR, Small SD, Glick S. Simulation-based medical education: an ethical imperative. Acad Med. 2003;78(8):783–8.

Chapter 13
The Role of Continuing Medical Education

Christina L. Jeng and Francine S. Yudkowitz

Introduction

There has been exceptional advancement in medical knowledge in the last century with an unprecedented growth in the scope of science that is the foundation of medicine. The total number of clinical trials has increased exponentially from 500 annually in the 1970s [1] to more than 10,000 since the late 1990s [2]. Funding from the National Institutes of Health (NIH) has appropriately increased from $300 in 1887 to $23.4 billion in 2002 [3] to almost $30 billion in 2011 [4].

This sudden increased advancement in the field of science has made it difficult for physicians to completely stay current. Students, residents, and faculty at academic institutions are in the prime position to acquire and apply this new information in their clinical practices. But because most practitioners do not work in environments that allow them to easily stay up-to-date, they may unintentionally offer patients medical care that is not in line with the current standard of care. It is especially difficult to maintain active learning in an environment of numerous responsibilities including clinical, administrative, educational, and personal obligations. To date, there are no published studies that evaluate the amount of time and the means necessary to maintain clinical competence throughout a physician's career.

What Is Continuing Medical Education?

Continuing Medical Education (CME) refers to the programs and resources designed to facilitate medical professionals in remaining up-to-date with emerging and developing science and technology in their respective fields. Because science and

---

C.L. Jeng, M.D. • F.S. Yudkowitz, M.D., F.A.A.P. (✉)
Department of Anesthesiology, Icahn School of Medicine at Mount Sinai,
1 Gustave L Levy Place, Box 1010, New York, NY 10029, USA
e-mail: christina.jeng@mountsinai.org; francine.yudkowitz@mountsinai.org

medicine are constantly evolving, physicians must be able to keep abreast of these changes and incorporate this new knowledge into their practice. CME programs are designed to ensure that this is occurring.

In the late 1920s, CME began in the United States when it was recognized that medical training of practicing physicians was inconsistent. Therefore, many medical schools began to create a system of continuing education after graduation. The first mandatory program was created by the specialty of urology in 1934. In 1957, the American Medical Association (AMA) published the first set of guidelines for reputable medical practice. By the 1960s, mandatory CME was widespread but the regulations varied by state. Physicians who completed 150 h of postgraduate medical training (PGME) within 3 years received an honorary diploma from the AMA. After much debate about the political predominance of the AMA in CME in the 1970s and 1980s, one unified association, the Accreditation Council for Continuing Medical Education (ACCME [5]), was created in 1981. ACCME is composed of seven entities who are the founding members: American Board of Medical Specialties (ABMS), American Hospital Association, AMA, Association of American Medical Colleges, Association for Hospital Medical Education, Council of Medical Specialty Societies, and Federation of State Medical Boards. However, the AMA continues to maintain an active role in CME [6] in that it defines which activities are eligible for CME credit.

The purpose of ACCME is to create a national accreditation system for CME providers that results in standardization of CME programs to ensure quality and transparency [7]. ACCME created a fairly rigorous process to ensure that the educational content of CME activities is valid and promote effective and safe health care. At the inception of ACCME, there were seven criteria called the Seven Essentials that accredited providers needed to follow. These seven criteria included the requirement of the program to identify the educational needs of their learners, create objectives for the activity, and to evaluate the effectiveness of their educational program. These seven criteria evolved over time to the present-day 22 criteria (Table 13.1) that were put into effect in 2006. Included in these criteria is the requirement to identify professional gaps (the difference between what physicians

Table 13.1 Accreditation criteria (as of this writing July 2013)

Criterion	
Essential area 1	Purpose and mission
1	The provider has a CME mission statement that includes all of the basic components (CME purpose, content areas, target audience, type of activities, expected results) with expected results articulated in terms of changes in competence, performance, or patient outcomes that will be the result of the program
Essential area 2	Education and planning
2	The provider incorporates into CME activities the educational needs (knowledge, competence, or performance) that underlie the professional practice gaps of their own learners

(continued)

Table 13.1 (continued)

Criterion	
3	The provider generates activities/educational interventions that are designed to change competence, performance, or patient outcomes as described in its mission statement
4	The provider generates activities/educational interventions around content that matches the learners' current or potential scope of professional activities
5	The provider chooses educational formats for activities/interventions that are appropriate for the setting, objectives, and desired results of the activity
6	The provider develops activities/educational interventions in the context of desirable physician attributes [e.g., Institute of Medicine (IOM) competencies, Accreditation Council for Graduate Medical Education (ACGME) competencies]
7	The provider develops activities/educational interventions independent of commercial interests
8	The provider appropriately manages commercial support
9	The provider maintains a separation of promotion from education
10	The provider actively promotes improvements in health care and NOT proprietary interests of a commercial interest
Essential area 3	Evaluation and improvement
11	The provider analyzes changes in learners (competence, performance, or patient outcomes) achieved as a result of the overall program's activities/educational interventions
12	The provider gathers data or information and conducts a program-based analysis on the degree to which the CME mission of the provider has been met through the conduct of CME activities/educational interventions
13	The provider identifies, plans, and implements the needed or desired changes in the overall program (e.g., planners, teachers, infrastructure, methods, resources, facilities, interventions) that are required to improve on ability to meet the CME mission
14	The provider demonstrates that identified program changes or improvements, that are required to improve on the provider's ability to meet the CME mission, are underway or completed
15	The provider demonstrates that the impacts of program improvements, that are required to improve on the provider's ability to meet the CME mission, are measured
	Accreditation with commendation
16	The provider operates in a manner that integrates CME into the process for improving professional practice
17	The provider utilizes non-education strategies to enhance change as an adjunct to its activities/educational interventions (e.g., reminders, patient feedback)
18	The provider identifies factors outside the provider's control that impact on patient outcomes
19	The provider implements educational strategies to remove, overcome, or address barriers to physician change
20	The provider builds bridges with other stakeholders through collaboration and cooperation
21	The provider participates within an institutional or system framework for quality improvement
22	The provider is positioned to influence the scope and content of activities/educational interventions

do and what they should be doing) of their learners, incorporating core competencies into their planning process (e.g., Institute of Medicine Core Competencies) and evaluating whether the program results in changing physician behavior. Six of the 22 criteria relate to the organization's engagement of the environment in which health care exists. For example, accredited providers are asked to identify physician barriers to change and address these barriers in their CME activities. Furthermore, as commercial entities as defined by ACCME ("any entity producing, marketing, re-selling, or distributing health care goods or services consumed by, or used on, patients") [8] began to support CME activities, the ACCME created policies to ensure that commercial bias was not introduced into CME activities by creating a Commercial Support Policy. CME providers are required to ensure that CME activities are free of bias from commercial entities. Additionally, all those in control of the educational content (e.g., planners, speakers) must disclose any financial relationship related to that activity. These disclosures must be vetted for potential conflict of interest that must be resolved prior to the start of the CME activity. Furthermore, all disclosures of financial relationships must be made to the learners so that they can decide for themselves whether bias was introduced into the presentation. Thus, the ultimate goal of ACCME is to ensure that CME activities across the United States are based on acceptable medical practice, contain valid content, free of commercial bias, and promote physician change that will ultimately improve patient outcomes.

To quantify physician participation in CME activities, the AMA developed the AMA Physician's Recognition Award (AMA PRA) of which there are two types, Category 1 and Category 2. Category 1 credits are earned by participating in CME activities by accredited providers, the AMA, or international programs recognized by the AMA. Category 2 credits are earned by individual physicians who apply to the AMA directly for participating in non-accredited activities. As a rule, for every hour of learning, one AMA PRA credit is awarded. Similar processes exist in the American Osteopathic Association [9] as well as in Canada by the Royal College of Physicians and Surgeons [10].

Presentation Formats

Currently, there are seven learning formats approved by the AMA that accredited providers can offer for *AMA PRA Category 1 Credit*™. Within all these formats, the AMA has set format-specific requirements that must be followed in order for credit to be awarded. The main goal in all of these formats is that the learner advances his/her knowledge, competence, or performance. These formats are as follows.

Live Activities

This is the most common form of CME activity offered. Although in the past this required the learner to attend in person, with the advent of teleconferencing and the Internet, learners do not have to travel to benefit from these offerings. This is especially beneficial in the current work environment where physicians are required to spend increasing time in clinical work. Educational formats also expanded from just large plenary session to include a multimodality format that includes any combination of the following: small group discussions, workshops, and simulation. One of the major benefits of a live activity is the ability to interact with identified experts and leaders in the field.

Enduring Materials

Enduring material is a CME activity that lasts for a specified period of time (e.g., 1 year). Initially, it consisted of monographs but with the advent of other media capabilities offerings now include DVD, podcasts, and archived webinars to name a few. Although this format does not allow interaction with the faculty, it does allow the physician to complete the activity at leisure. As pointed out above, this is a great advantage for physicians today who have ever increasing clinical commitments. Commonly, a posttest with a minimum passing grade is utilized to assess whether the learner achieved the desired result from participation in this CME activity.

Enduring materials may also be presented as part of a monthly publication, requiring either an annual subscription or a fee on a monthly basis. Typically these programs offer credit at a substantially lower rate than is generated by meeting attendance (approximately 2 credits per month). An honor system requires that subscribers report the length of time it required to complete the learning assignment (but usually not to exceed 2 h) and complete a post-test. These programs can often be completed electronically and the credit received immediately acknowledged. However, any programs so offered must be accredited by a recognized accrediting facility and undergo the same rigorous review, usually on a biannual basis.

Journal-Based

An article in a peer-reviewed professional journal identified by a CME provider prior to publication is eligible for CME credit. As with enduring materials, an assessment of the learner's achievement is necessary for credits to be awarded.

Test Item Writing

A physician who participates in preparing high-stakes examinations (e.g., board exam) or peer-reviewed self-assessment activities is eligible to receive CME credit. The basis by which this activity is eligible for CME credit is that the physician learned while researching and preparing the content of the product and will be able to respond to questions related to the topics researched.

Manuscript Review for Journals

This format involves critical review of an original manuscript submitted for publication in a journal that is included in MEDLINE and requires multiple reviewers. The expectation is that the physician will need to review the literature and be knowledgeable about the evidence supporting the educational content of the manuscript.

Performance Improvement CME

Performance Improvement (PI) CME involves a three-stage process. In the first stage, the learner assesses an aspect of his/her practice against identified performance measures. The second stage consists of implementing an intervention to improve performance. After an appropriate interval of time has passed, the third stage begins and the learner reassesses his/her practice using the same performance measure used in stage 1. A total of 20 CME credits are awarded at completion of all three stages. However, if the learner only completes one or two stages, he/she is entitled to 5 credits for each stage completed. Recently, this format was included in the Maintenance of Certification in Anesthesiology (MOCA) requirement.

Internet Point-of-Care Learning

As with PI CME, this format involves self-direction by the learner. Learners identify a topic relevant to their practice, pose a clinical question, and conduct an online search to answer that question. Learners are expected to reflect on what they learned and how it applies to their practice.

Physicians participating in educational activities not certified by an accredited provider can apply to the AMA for Category 2 credits. The same rigorous standards apply to these activities in that they have to meet the AMA's definition of CME. The physician needs to identify how this learning experience related to his/her practice. Some examples of activities eligible for Category 2 credits are teaching residents or medical students, consulting with peers and medical experts, self-assessment activities, medical writing, and reading authoritative medical literature.

Available CME Activities

With the multitude of CME activities offered every year, physicians may find it difficult to identify a CME activity that meets all their needs. To this end, the American Society of Anesthesiologists (ASA) maintains on their website a list of offered CME activities (Anesthesiology-Related Meetings and Events, www.asahq.org/For-Members/Education-and-Events/Calendar-of-Events.aspx). Although this is an ASA site, other accredited providers can submit their CME activities for inclusion on this site. When submitting, the accredited provider is asked to categorize the activity by date, location, type of activity, and educational content. The benefit of this website to physicians is that they can search by keyword for a CME activity that fits their needs. Searchable parameters include date (month, year), location (state, country), type (live, webinar, simulation, etc.), and content (cardiac, ambulatory, pediatric, board review, etc.).

In the field of anesthesiology, there are four major recognized CME activities: the ASA Annual Meeting, the International Anesthesia Research Society (IARS) Annual Meeting, the New York State Society of Anesthesiologists (NYSSA) Postgraduate Assembly (PGA), and the California Society of Anesthesiologists (CSA) Annual Meeting. These four meetings each occur over a 4–5-day period and offer a large number of sessions in a variety of educational formats (e.g., plenary, problem-based learning discussions, small group sessions, workshops) encompassing topics from the complete spectrum of anesthesia practice. This allows the attendees to select sessions in the format of their preference in a concentrated period of time that meets their needs. A physician attending these meetings is able to earn a large number of CME credits at one time.

Smaller state and subspecialty societies also have their own annual meetings, but they usually occur over a shorter period of time (usually over 1–3 days). Subspecialty societies provide more focused CME activities. For example, the American Society of Regional Anesthesia provides CME activities related to only regional anesthesia.

Another major CME offering are review courses. These activities aim to be comprehensive and tend to have many sessions based on the American Board of Anesthesiology (ABA) core curriculum. Although these activities are directed to those preparing for the board examination or recertification process, many physicians attend these meetings as a "refresher course." These review courses tend to be over 3–5 days and offer a large number of CME credits.

CME credits can be obtained through self-study. The advantage of this method versus live activities is that the learner doesn't have to travel and can participate according to their schedule. For example, the ASA offers Self-Education and Evaluation (SEE) and Anesthesiology Continuing Education (ACE) programs, which are offered to members for a fee. The SEE and ACE programs each provide up to 60 CME credits annually and both are required to satisfy MOCA requirements.

Reasons for CME Activities

Lifelong Learning

Physicians are committed to lifelong learning because the practice of medicine is continually evolving and changing. Therefore, the most important reason for participation in CME activities is for personal enhancement and education.

As physicians, we strive to increase our knowledge and competence of proven new treatments and technology and apply these to our daily practice. In the end, this results in better quality and safer care of our patients and improved patient outcomes.

Licensure, Credentialing, and Privileging

Although physicians participated voluntarily in CME activities as part of personal improvement, regulatory agencies decided to mandate minimum yearly CME credit requirements. For example, in order to maintain state licensure, a minimum number of earned CME credits are required. The number of CME credits required, however, varies from state to state. Furthermore, certain states have further delineated this requirement to obtaining a set number of CME credits in certain areas (e.g., infection control, child abuse).

Hospitals also incorporate CME credit requirement into their credentialing and privileging process. Some hospitals may place additional conditions on these CME credit requirements such as the number of credits that must be obtained at the home institution.

Finally, malpractice insurance companies have also instituted requirements for specific CME activities related to the risk reduction of malpractice suits.

Maintenance of Certification in Anesthesiology

In 1999, The American Board of Medical Specialties (ABMS) initiated the concept of Maintenance of Certification (MOC). The intent of MOC is to ensure that physicians keep current on advances in their field of practice, develop better practice systems, and make a commitment to lifelong learning. Basically, all medical specialties are involved in this program; however, the specific requirements to fulfill MOC are determined by the individual specialty board. Although the intention of the MOC program is honorable, there are no studies to show that it improves any measurable outcome.

The ABA, a member of the ABMS, is committed to the highest quality in clinical outcomes and patient safety. As of 2000, time-limited board certification was instituted and all physicians graduating from that time forth are required to participate in the MOCA process. Physicians completing board certification prior to 2000 who do not have time-limited certification are encouraged to participate in the MOCA process. MOCA is a four-part process (Table 13.2) that must be completed in a 10-year period. Failure to complete all four parts results in certification expiration. The individual components and requirements are constantly evolving and the diplomate is urged to refer to the ABA website for the most current information on the requirements for MOCA completion.

Part 1 consists of *assessment of professional standing*. Maintaining an active medical license fulfills this requirement.

Table 13.2 Maintenance of certification in anesthesiology (as of this writing July 2013)

Part	Description	Requirements
Part 1	Assessment of professional standing	Maintenance of medical licensure
Part 2	Lifelong learning and self-assessment	Minimum of 250 *CME AMA PRA Category 1 Credit*™
		No more than 60 credits per year
		Minimum of 90 credits of ABA-approved self-assessment CME as follows:
		ASA's ACE program (60 credits)
		ASA's SEE program (60 credits)
		ASA self-assessment module—pain medicine (30 credits)
		ASA self-assessment module—critical care medicine (30 credits)
		Minimum of 20 credits of ABA-approved patient safety CME as follows:
		ASA's fundamental of patient safety (10 credits) *required*
		Additional 10 credits of ABA-approved patient safety CME activities
Part 3	Cognitive test	Taken years 7–10 of the cycle
		May take it twice a year
		If not passed at 10 years, certification expires
Part 4	Periodic assessment of practice performance	Case evaluation and simulation
		One activity to be completed during years 1–5 and the other during years 6–10

Part 2 consists of *lifelong learning and self-assessment.* CME is recognized as an important component of the MOCA process. A minimum of 250 *AMA PRA Category 1 Credit*™ must be earned by the end of the 10-year cycle. These CME credits are further parsed into a minimum of 90 CME credits for self-assessment activities and a minimum of 20 CME credits in patient safety that are pre-approved by the ABA. Self-assessment activities are meant to aid the diplomate in determining their level of knowledge, while the traditional CME activities are meant to increase knowledge, competence, and performance. It is expected that the diplomate will achieve improvement in the six core competencies: medical knowledge, patient care, practice-based learning and improvement, professionalism, interpersonal and communication skills, and systems-based practice.

Part 3 is the *cognitive examination* that can only be taken during years 7–10 of the cycle. The examination can be taken twice a year starting in the seventh year. Failure to pass the examination results in certification expiration at the end of the 10-year cycle.

Part 4, *periodic assessment of practice performance*, has undergone the greatest change over time. At the time of this writing, to fulfill this component of MOCA, a case evaluation and simulation course must be completed. One must be completed during years 1–5 and the other during years 6–10. The order of completion does not matter.

Funding

In the past, the majority of funding for CME activities was provided by commercial entities in the health care field. However, in recent years the trend has been away from commercial funding because of the perceived potential for influence on physicians to use a particular drug or equipment in their practice that did not meet evidence-based scrutiny. According to the ACCME, an accredited provider must ensure that the CME activities sponsored remain free of the control of commercial interests. Furthermore, all educational content must promote improvements or quality in health care and be free of commercial bias.

As greater restrictions are imposed on commercial funding, the financial burden of acquiring CME credits falls on the individual physician or their employer. Even when the individual anesthesiologist bears the financial burden, their employer still needs to allow time away from practice [11]. With the advent of MOCA, a considerable financial burden is now placed on the diplomate in order to complete all four components. But as yet, there is no evidence to support that MOCA actually improves patient care or outcomes. It will take several years to be able to document improved outcome, fewer lawsuits, or a decrease in reported critical incidents.

References

1. Chassin MR, Galvin RW. The urgent need to improve health care quality. Institute of Medicine National Roundtable on Health Care Quality. JAMA. 1998;280(11):1000–5.
2. Krall RL. US Clinical research. Presentation at the Institute of Medicine workshop on transforming clinical research in the United States. Washington, DC; Oct 2009.
3. National Institutes of Health. National Institutes of Health: an overview. http://www.nih.gov/about/NIHoverview.html
4. National Institutes of Health. NIH budget history. http://report.nih.gov/nihdatabook
5. http://www.accme.org. Accessed 20 July 2013.
6. Josseran L, Chaperon J. History of continuing medical education in the United States. Presse Med. 2001;30(10):493–7.
7. Wentz DK. Continuing medical education at a crossroads. JAMA. 1990;264:2425–6.
8. http://www.accme.org/requirements/accreditation-requirements-cme-providers/policies-and-definitions/definition-commercial-interest. Accessed 23 July 2014.
9. Reuther GA. AOA continuing medical education. J Am Osteopath Assoc. 1990;90:1020–6.
10. Parboosingh JT, Gondocz ST. The maintenance of competence program of the Royal College of Physicians and Surgeons of Canada. JAMA. 1993;270:1093.
11. Toghill PJ. Continuing medical education for physicians. J R Coll Physicians. 1994;28:155–6.

Chapter 14
Multidisciplinary Teaching: The Interaction of the Specialties

Michael Yarborough, Brian McClure, and Santiago Gomez

Why Anesthesiology?

As pressure to provide better patient care at less cost increases, all specialties are involved [1]. When we are faced with the question, "Are there ways that we can improve our anesthesiology training?" the answer appears to be yes. When one looks at historical anesthesia training which has involved trainees who were taught in a traditional apprenticeship paradigm, research has identified poor, unsupervised practice [2]. In addition, there is an increased incidence of anesthesia-related morbidity and mortality occurring in the beginning of the academic year [3–5]. Another argument for a need to relook at our traditional training comes from the considerable body of evidence documenting the negative effects of sleep deprivation on both trainees and staff. In response to this evidence, many jurisdictions, over the past decade, have mandated reduced working hours, which, in turn, have resulted in concerns of decreased training opportunities and lack of continuity of medical care [6, 7]. These changes force us to reconsider how we are teaching medical education.

Bould et al. posed the following questions regarding the challenges faced by the twenty-first-century anesthesiology educator. As a specialty, how can we ensure that residents are trained adequately to deal with the ever increasing complexity of the modern healthcare system while simultaneously structuring training programs to minimize the fatigue shown to lead to medical error and burn out? Is it possible to improve the efficiency of training programs so that residents learn more in a shorter period of time? Is it possible to reduce the risks to patients inherent in anesthesiology training, especially in earlier phases of learning? How can we assess the

---

M. Yarborough, M.D. (✉) • B. McClure, M.D. • S. Gomez, M.D.
Department of Anesthesiology, Tulane School of Medicine,
1430 Tulane Avenue, SL-4, New Orleans, LA 70112-2699, USA
e-mail: myarboro@tulane.edu; brianmcclure@yahoo.com

cost-effectiveness and efficacy of new technologies for use in medical education? What is the most effective means to teach residents the knowledge base and skill sets for rare events so they can retain the acquired skills for when they are needed [8]? Questions such as these point us in a direction away from the traditional training approaches that we have historically embraced. When reviewing different approaches for successful training, multidisciplinary education becomes not only more acceptable but more desirable.

Upon simple reflection of the specialty of anesthesiology, it becomes glaringly apparent just how integral multidisciplinary education should be to the anesthesia curriculum. Anesthesiologists work intimately with various specialists in an ever-growing number of fields. In the spectrum of practice, there are physicians, nurses, and technicians, just to name a few. Each individual brings to the table not only a level of knowledge that is unique but a depth and complexity that stems from the patient comorbidities, surgical intricacies, and medical technology. The goal should be the ability for this team to interact and communicate seamlessly about the patient without becoming specialists in each other's fields. However, often, this is not the case. Hopefully, through effective multidisciplinary education, this goal can be achieved.

One of the aspects of anesthesiology, perhaps more than any other specialty, is the reliance on teamwork. It is extremely rare for an anesthesiologist to work in isolation. The hospital-based practice of anesthesiology, whether it be working in the operating room, intensive care unit, or a more isolated location, is strongly reliant on a team mentality. In the operating room, the anesthesiologist could be working in unison with a litany of potential participants including the surgeon, the scrub technician, the circulating nurse, radiology technician, medical device representative, monitoring specialist, nurse anesthetist, or anesthesiology resident to name a few. The ability to not only "play nice," but interact and direct the team if necessary, is paramount to a successful patient experience. Poor teamwork in a crisis situation could potentially result in catastrophe, but at a minimum will surely result in less than desirable results. One of the challenges of anesthesiology training is developing a curriculum that teaches solid team concepts and augments the positive aspects of successful team dynamics. Multidisciplinary education has been at the forefront of such developments for a long time in the aviation industry and has become more accepted and prominent in multiple other industries [9, 10].

Patient safety is a wonderful example of the need to adapt with multidisciplinary education. Safety in healthcare is no longer delivered by individual professionals. Safety is a team topic that crosses the boundaries of all professions in healthcare. Patient safety has not only been an immense concern for anesthesiologists, but anesthesiology has been a model for patient safety at the local, national, and international levels. Patient safety training is a multidisciplinary topic and enterprise, which requires anesthesiologists to cooperate with safety experts from different fields (e.g., psychologists, educators, human factor experts) [11]. Through multidisciplinary education, anesthesiology can continue to be the leader in the development of patient safety initiatives.

Definitions

As we begin discussing multidisciplinary education we need to ask, "What is multidisciplinary education?" If one were to ask different educators for a definition, one would almost certainly end up with a great number of varied answers. Although most would be somewhat similar, there would still be significant variations. Over the past half century, the medical literature has used the terms multidisciplinary, interdisciplinary, multiprofessional, and interprofessional interchangeably [1]. One common distinction is that multidisciplinary education suggests that two or more specialties learn together, whereas interdisciplinary education additionally implies the goal of promoting cooperative practice [12]. One task force at Saint Louis University Health Sciences Center, when faced with developing a methodology of teaching interdisciplinary education in the primary care practice, defined interdisciplinary education as a process of teaching health professional students the knowledge, attitudes, and skills needed for the interdisciplinary practice of healthcare [13]. The United Kingdom Centre for the Advancement of Interprofessional Education has defined interprofessional education as follows: "Interprofessional education is those occasions when members (or students) of two or more professions learn with, from and about one another to improve collaboration and the quality of care" [14]. The World Health Organization, in 2010, defined interprofessional education as occurring "when two or more professions learn about, from and with each other to enable effective collaboration and improve health outcomes" [1]. These definitions should help focus the discussion of interdisciplinary education as it relates to teaching anesthesiology.

History

As stated previously, multiprofessional education has been evolving over the past half century. A brief historical assessment of the advancements in multidisciplinary education is beneficial to understanding where we are today. It may even point to where we might be headed in the not too distant future.

In the 1960s, authors began to emerge in the relatively new field of interdisciplinary education. Those in education recommended or commented on interdisciplinary educational approaches while those in practice provided a historical, clinical, or sociological context for subsequent educational opportunities. The importance of teamwork was discussed while successful and unsuccessful student, faculty, and practitioner experiences were reviewed [13].

The 1970s saw diverse attempts to address the issue of multidisciplinary education and practice. Models to describe current and future directions of multidisciplinary education and practice were developed. The models of this decade were aimed at restructuring health professional education. Internationally, the literature of the 1970s displayed growing interest in interdisciplinary education, practice, and research issues [13].

Two notable developments in the field of multidisciplinary education occurred in the 1980s. Concepts were clarified and the contrast between interdisciplinary development between the United States and the rest of the world became more clear. While the rest of the world was covering broader clinical interests, the United States was following funding in the field of gerontology. In addition, multidisciplinary education models dealt with concrete issues of identifying institutional characteristics critical to success and defining terms and practice issues [13].

It wasn't until the 1990s that interdisciplinary education and practice outcomes became a focus for research. Courses that were developed during this time were eclectic and innovative. There was an increase in differentiation among interdisciplinary education models. These were remarkable for their creativity [13]. As an example, a three-phase multidisciplinary model was developed. The phases included (1) introduction to interdisciplinary practice/issues, (2) interdisciplinary problem-based learning sessions, and (3) multidisciplinary team assessment of a client [15].

The turn of the century saw the continued progress of multidisciplinary education and practice as a global movement. Over the past decade plus, interprofessional and multidisciplinary education has assumed a place as a key theme in the medical education literature [8]. There are continued efforts for evidence to back the support that multidisciplinary education has garnered. In addition, a recent Cochrane review suggested that interprofessional education can improve healthcare processes and outcomes [16]. As we continue the progression, we are seeing the drive for interprofessional education to present the logistic and organizational/cultural issues involved in gathering different professional groups with the ultimate goal of improving quality of care through coordinated curriculum design [8].

Differing Levels of Multiprofessional Education

Some believe that the question with multiprofessional education is not whether it is effective or not, but under what circumstances can this educational strategy be effective. Harden proposed taking a three-dimensional approach to assisting with the success of multidisciplinary education. The three dimensions included:

1. The context in which the multiprofessional education is to be applied (including the phase or stage of education, category of student, and the educational format)
2. The curriculum goals (expected outcomes)
3. The approach to multiprofessional education to be adopted (multidisciplinary education is not one entity, but a continuum) [17]

We need to examine these dimensions a little closer to gain a greater understanding of his proposal.

Many discussions regarding the success of multidisciplinary education regarding the context of education have focused on the difference between the basic education level student and the advanced education student. While this has traditionally been described with subjects other than anesthesiology, it can easily be translated into the level of training of anesthesiologist from medical student to staff anesthesiologist. Some argue that multidisciplinary education should occur at an advanced level allowing the basic learner to develop their own identity prior to being exposed to the influences of other professions. Others, however, propose that there are powerful incentives for moving multidisciplinary education to the early stages of training. These include education occurring prior to being imprinted with potential prejudices of one's specialty. What appears to matter most is incorporating an approach that is appropriate to that phase of education [17].

Other aspects of the context important in developing successful multidisciplinary education include the setting, the topic, and the learning approach. The setting is often overlooked in initial planning, but must be considered. Where the teaching takes place is extremely important and must be planned properly. One does not want to put the effort into developing a solid multidisciplinary education experience only to be undermined by an inappropriate setting. On the issue of the topic, it is usually self-explanatory. Sometimes it is a subject that is chosen and developed by the organizer of the educational experience and sometimes it is assigned to the educator. Either way the planner must work to incorporate the proper approach to make the effort successful. The learning approach can be in different contexts. Examples include small groups, lectures, distance learning, and problem-based learning [17]. Just as the setting can undermine a successful experience, the approach must be carefully selected to ensure success.

The curriculum goals, that is, what one hopes to achieve with multidisciplinary educational event, must be clear and achievable. While most common goals are collaborative skills and the ability to work as a team, there can be an immeasurable number of goal choices. Careful reflection on just what one is trying to achieve with the educational experience is necessary if successful education is to be achieved. The choice of the most appropriate approach to multidisciplinary education will vary with the goals or outcomes desired [17].

There are many varied approaches that can be utilized in the execution of multidisciplinary education. Just as there are multiple approaches to education and all can be effective, choosing the most appropriate approach will assist with achieving the greatest result. When one looks at these approaches, it becomes noticeable that there is really a continuum of educational experiences. Harden has described different approaches to integrated teaching and learning with 11 steps as points in his continuum between discipline or subject-based teaching on one end of the spectrum and integrated or multidisciplinary teaching at the other end. The steps that he has delineated are as follows [17]:

1. Isolation—No contact between different professions.
2. Awareness—Each profession has awareness of the others role but there is no formal collaboration.
3. Consultation—Discussion between the different professions, but the program for each profession remains separate and distinct.

4. Nesting—An effort is made to provide students in one profession with a perspective or understanding or another profession, but there is no joint or shared teaching.
5. Temporal coordination—It is the first step towards joint teaching and involves changes in the timetable so that two or more professions can be scheduled for a similar experience at the same time.
6. Shared teaching—Adds the interaction between the different professions as part of the scheduled teaching program.
7. Correlation—Emphasis remains on uniprofessional education; however, there are scheduled regular and well-defined multiprofessional sessions.
8. Complimentary—Emphasis on both uniprofessional and multiprofessional education, each complimenting each other.
9. Multiprofessional education—Emphasis on multiprofessional education with little devoted to uniprofessional education.
10. Interprofessional education—No distinction between the different professions of the students with each student looking at the subject from the perspective of other professions as well as their own.
11. Transprofessional education—Multiprofessional education occurring in the clinical practice of medicine.

As one can tell with this evolution of educational concepts from an isolationist approach to a fully integrated, within multidisciplinary education, there are endless options in choosing the most appropriate approach to an educational goal. As such, one must choose the approach that is felt to provide the best advantage in order to succeed.

Driving Forces

There are a number of forces or challenges that can drive the project of multidisciplinary education towards either success or failure. Knowledge of these forces is important when one is attempting to maximize the potential for success while undertaking the challenge of developing a multidisciplinary education project. One would want to lean on and even highlight the positive forces while minimizing the negative obstacles that could be encountered.

Positive Forces

It is widely assumed that "learning together" (effectively) is a necessary and sufficient precondition for "working together" (effectively) [12]. Most would argue that if individuals are aiming to work together as a solid team, then they must train (or learn) together as a team. Just as no one would expect the New England Patriots to practice individually and still maintain the exceptional performance on the field that has become expected, one should view multidisciplinary education as one of the pieces (or practices) leading up to the big game. In order to function as smoothly as possible, we must work together to gain understanding of not only the common goal but each team members expectations in order to achieve that goal.

Initially, in order to have any chance for success, both staff and students must be convinced of the rational for the inclusion of multidisciplinary education. In addition to buying into the approach, using principles of adult learning is extremely valuable allowing multidisciplinary education to be well received. Additionally, authenticity from the learning experience is greatly needed due to the unique nature of multidisciplinary education. Finally, customization so that the educational process reflects the reality of practice acts as a mechanism for positive outcomes [14].

"Product Champions" have the power to be the sole determinant in regard to the success or failure of an educational enterprise. "Product Champions" are individuals who have the unique ability and the energy to champion the end goal. Just as in any educational project, "product champions" are a huge force towards the success of multidisciplinary education objectives [12]. In many cases, the success of an initiative is attributed to one particular individual's contribution. That individual has the charisma, drive, and energy to ensure the success of the project. It must also be noted that if that individual moves on, this can hinder any further propagation of the initiative as the driving force behind the success is lost.

Course organizers and students need to develop a common sense of purpose and a clear understanding of the rational for multidisciplinary education [12]. The type of student, for example, can make a large difference. More mature and experienced learners appear to be more favorably disposed towards multidisciplinary education than younger, less experienced learners [18]. Just as the student is important in ensuring success in multidisciplinary education, the teacher can be paramount. One study found that the "quality of the supervision was the most important contribution to student satisfaction" [19]. The common belief that a great teacher will be successful no matter what the circumstances may be true, but in order for all teachers to be successful with multidisciplinary education, one must institute the proper preparatory platform for teachers to educate utilizing this approach. Whether it is through a faculty development program or individual preparation, it is key for the teacher to be well prepared to take on the challenge of teaching multidisciplinary education. Studies have found that some teachers felt unprepared for facilitating interprofessional groups of medical, nursing, and dental students in seminar discussions and that there were "staff training implications if educators are required to act as interprofessional role models" [20, 21].

Interprofessional education normally occurs as the result of a desire to improve patient outcomes or service delivery. Usually, this is through improvement of interprofessional collaboration (teamwork) [14]. This can be driven from the healthcare provider realizing a need for improvement and taking the initiative to finding a way to establish multidisciplinary educational approach to finding a solution. This bottom-up stimulus is one example of how these initiatives can occur. Another example is via a top-down approach often from someone of higher authority mandating a need to produce results. A term that has been developed in this scenario is "transition driver." A "transition driver" is often an educator or clinical manager who acts via a top-down call to initiate, develop, and deliver interprofessional education [14].

Obstacles to Success

Skepticism regarding the effectiveness of multidisciplinary education is diverse and frequently encountered. Especially in a specialty, such as anesthesiology, where we rely heavily on evidence-based standards to guide our practice of medicine, the lack of intense scientific studies proving the merit of multidisciplinary medicine fuels those who want to doubt or obstruct this teaching modality. The difficulty in performing our gold standard, the randomized controlled trials, in examining educational approaches leaves a dearth of information that many rely heavily on before changing their ways. The variability in teachers and learners makes the randomization extremely questionable. In addition, with true randomization, oftentimes the control group feels deprived of improved materials and strategies. When outcome improvements are measured, they are often obscured by so many variables that occur with such a process that this results in blunted effect.

Another aspect that often causes concern or lack of support is the ambiguity of the terms utilized. As described earlier, the terms "multidisciplinary," "interdisciplinary," "multiprofessional," and "interprofessional" have been used interchangeably for a considerable period of time now [12]. This terminology confusion has led to decreased support due to difficulty researching articles and methods (requirements to search the multiple terms can be time consuming) and a decrease in familiarity of what is one continuum of education and not four distinct processes.

In addition, some healthcare providers feel an overwhelming need to establish, and maintain, professional identities. They perceive the institution of multidisciplinary education as a threat to their identity and thus are reluctant to fully support these measures. Their need to maintain professional identity, standards, and value systems pervades much of the data that is available [12].

The timing of such an educational event is a constant threat to the success of the program. The organization and implementation of multidisciplinary courses make heavy demands on staff in terms of personal commitment and effective teamwork. Perhaps, the biggest challenge is actually getting the personnel (from different departments, faculties, institutions, etc.) together. In a study of interprofessional education for clinical skills, Tucker et al. reported that "timetabling the sessions to identify times when all students were free was problematic" [22]. Another similarly timed study found that the most significant barrier to success was the practical issues of shift and timetable incompatibility [21].

Other obstacles that may be encountered include such logistical challenges of finding adequate meeting room space (both large room and multiple small rooms). Many professionals want equal representation in the education process in both the faculty role and the learner role. This can be a cumbersome obstacle that sometimes can only be overcome through time-consuming, personal coaxing. Access to library and IT facilities can be another issue, especially if large numbers of students are involved [12].

Knowledge of the factors that can either hinder or promote the success of a multidisciplinary education is invaluable. Maximizing the positives and minimizing the negatives is a recipe for success in any enterprise, but is especially necessary when attempting a new educational technique. Through proper manipulation of variables, it is easier to ensure success during planning.

Positive Results

When trying to plan for success with the restraints presented previously, one would like to be inspired by knowledge that they are not traveling through uncharted territory. While this process of evolution towards the embracing of multidisciplinary education has been a slow, tedious transformation that has been occurring over the past half century, there are some good examples of positive research which can be inspiring. Minehart et al. reported of a successful multidisciplinary education opportunity revolving around the management of a surgical maternal crisis [23]. In this example, a simulation experience was analyzed for communication aspects between anesthesiologists and obstetricians, and, upon review, the interactions could be improved upon through a multidisciplinary education experience involving communication styles and possibly help teams arrive more efficiently at jointly managed clinical plans in crisis situations.

Palliative Medicine is an area that has emerged as an area that could be utilized as an example for anesthesiology as a means to incorporate multidisciplinary education into the foundations of training. Vissers et al. reported on the need for palliative medicine to incorporate a multidisciplinary approach in its teaching. Due to complexity of care for incurable patients, it is felt that the multidisciplinary approach is a prerequisite for balancing curative and palliative intervention options. Optional functioning as a team is key to proper patient care [24]. Direct correlations can be drawn with the complexity of anesthesiology and the complex care/teamwork required to care for our patients effectively.

Another example of works in progress involves the University of Washington School of Medicine, who published their success story in 2013 [25]. After assessing the educational process of their medical students in relation to pain, they felt that their curriculum was lacking in producing the desired results. As such, they redesigned their course to cover a 4-year time interval which increased the required teaching time from 6 to 25 h. The curriculum was redesigned under the oversight of "Pain Theme Committee" composed of multispecialty educators and clinicians including anesthesiologists, internists, neurosurgeons, psychologists, and pediatric psychologists. Through these measures the educational expectations of the medical students have been raised, and the opportunities for elective pain education courses have increased by 80 % [25].

Summary

Anesthesiology training has been slowly evolving over its history. Upon review of the techniques and traditions that are currently used for training our future anesthesiologists, it becomes apparent that educators need to continue to adapt and improvise in order to better educate our residents. One technique that should be added to the educational repertoire is multidisciplinary education. The need to practice in a multispecialty arena and rely on multiple professionals to assist with our daily success has come to define what anesthesiologists do. Through multidisciplinary education, anesthesiologists should be better prepared to flourish in the current and future healthcare environment. An opportunity to train with our fellow practitioners should break down some of the historical barriers between different professionals allowing for better patient care. Although the research is still being done on the effectiveness of multidisciplinary education, this tool appears to be an extremely powerful modality which should be implemented. With proper preparation and selection, this opportunity for education could bring powerful, long-term results. Most importantly, the final aspect is that the people who will experience the greatest benefit from such an enterprise are the ones we care about most, the patients that we have the honor of caring for every day.

References

1. Kveraga R, Jones SB. Improving quality through multidisciplinary education. Anesthesiol Clin. 2011;29:99–110.
2. Friedman Z, Siddiqui N, Katznelson R, Devito I, Davies S. Experience is not enough: repeated breaches in epidural anesthesia aseptic technique by novice operators despite improved skill. Anesthesiology. 2008;108:914–20.
3. Haller G, Myles PS, Taffe PV, Perneger T, Wu CL. Rate of undesirable events at beginning of academic year: retrospective cohort study. BMJ. 2009;339:b3974.
4. Nash R. The "killing season": does inexperience cost lives? Lancet. 2009;374:1313–4.
5. Jen M, Bottle A, Majeed A, Bell D, Aylin P. Early in-hospital mortality following trainee doctors' first day at work. PLoS One. 2009;4:7103.
6. Fernandez E, Williams DG. Training and the European Working Time Directive: a 7 year review of paediatric anaesthetic training caseload data. Br J Anaesth. 2009;103:566–9.
7. Sim DJ, Wrigley SR, Harris S. Effects of the European Working Time Directive on anaesthetic training in the United Kingdom. Anaesthesia. 2004;59:781–4.
8. Bould MD, Naik VN, Hamstra SJ. Review article: new directions in medical education related to anesthesiology and perioperative medicine. Can J Anaesth. 2012;59:136–50.
9. Sundar E, Sundar S, Pawlowski J, Blum R, Feinstein D, Pratt S. Crew resource management and team training. Anesthesiol Clin. 2007;25:283–300.
10. Hunt EA, Shilkofski NA, Stavroudis TA, Nelson KL. Simulation: translation to improved team performance. Anesthesiol Clin. 2007;25:301–19.
11. Rall M, van Gessel E, Staender S. Education, teaching and training in patient safety. Best Pract Res Clin Anaesthesiol. 2011;25(2):251–62.
12. Pirrie A, Hamilton S, Wilson V. Multidisciplinary education: some issues and concerns. Educ Res. 1999;41(3):301–14.

13. Lavin MA, Ruebling I, Banks R, Block L, Counte M, Furman G, Miller P, Reese C, Viehmann V, Holt J. Interdisciplinary health professional education: a historical review. Adv Health Sci Educ Theory Pract. 2001;6:25–47.
14. Hammick M, Freeth D, Koppel I, Reeves S, Barr H. A best evidence systematic review of interprofessional education: BEME Guide no. 9. Med Teach. 2007;29:735–51.
15. Lary MJ, Lavigne SE, Muma RD, Jones SE, Hoeft HJ. Breaking down barriers: multidisciplinary education model. J Allied Health. 1997;26(2):63–9.
16. Zwarenstein M, Goldman J, Reeves S. Interprofessional collaboration: effects of practice-based interventions on professional practice and healthcare outcomes. Cochrane Database Syst Rev. 2009;(3):CD000072.
17. Harden RM. AMEE guide No. 12: multiprofessional education: Part I—effective multiprofessional education: a three-dimensional perspective. Med Teach. 1998;20(5):402–8.
18. Tunstall-Pedoe S, Rink E, Hilton S. Student attitudes to undergraduate interprofessional education. J Interprof Care. 2003;17:161–72.
19. Ponzer S, Hylin U, Kusoffsky A, Lauffs M, Lonka K, Mattiasson A, Nordstrom G. Interprofessional training in the context of clinical practice: goals and students' perceptions on clinical education wards. Med Educ. 2004;38:727–36.
20. Reeves S. Community-based interprofessional education for medical, nursing and dental students. Health Soc Care Community. 2000;4:269–76.
21. Morison S, Boohan M, Jenkins J, Moutray M. Facilitating undergraduate interprofessional learning in healthcare: comparing classroom and clinical learning for nursing and medical students. Learn Health Soc Care. 2003;2:92–104.
22. Tucker K, Wakefield A, Boggis C, Lawson M, Roberts T, Gooch J. Learning together: clinical skills teaching for medical and nursing students. Med Educ. 2003;37:630–7.
23. Minehart RD, Pian-Smith MCM, Walzer TB, Gardner R, Rudolph JW, Simon R, Raemer DB. Speaking across the drapes: communication strategies of anesthesiologists and obstetricians during a simulated maternal crisis. Simul Healthc. 2012;7(3):166–70.
24. Vissers KCP, van den Brand MWM, Jacobs J, Groot M, Veldhoven C, Verhagen C, Hasselaar J, Engels Y. Palliative medicine update: a multidisciplinary approach. Pain Pract. 2013;13(7):576–88. [epub ahead of print].
25. Tauben DJ, Loeser JD. Pain education at the University of Washington School of Medicine. J Pain. 2013;14(5):431–7.

Chapter 15
Research in Education

Robert Fallar, Reena Karani, and Erica Friedman

Medical Education Research

Research in medical education is critical for demonstrating the effectiveness of educational interventions and for identifying new methods of teaching and assessment. Education research can facilitate the careful and systematic approach to educational innovations, bridge the gap between education theory and practice, and support policy changes. Research also allows us to study new advances in science and technology in order to clarify their benefit and identify how to best use this information to facilitate learning. Taking a scholarly approach to education research allows others to determine the value of an intervention. Additionally, given that we are often tasked with improving the efficiency and effectiveness of medical education, studying the impact of teaching and learning approaches provides important data to guide such improvements.

R. Fallar, M.S. (✉)
The Mount Sinai Medical Center, New York, NY, USA

Department of Medicine, Icahn School of Medicine at Mount Sinai,
1425 Madison Avenue, New York, NY 10029, USA
e-mail: robert.fallar@mssm.edu

R. Karani, M.D., M.H.P.E.
Department of Medical Education, Icahn School of Medicine at Mount Sinai,
Room 1330, 1468 Madison Avenue, New York, NY 10029, USA
e-mail: reena.karani@mssm.edu

E. Friedman, M.D., F.A.C.P.
Sophie Davis School of Biomedical Education, City College,
City University of New York, New York, NY, USA

Why Should You Do Education Research?

Increasingly, academic medical centers are recognizing the importance of education research and have created clinician educator tracks which facilitate academic promotion based upon education scholarship. The Association of American Medical Colleges (AAMC) Educational Working Group on Educational Scholarship developed a series of documents that describe the definition, peer review, publication, and recognition of educational scholarship in health education and illustrate how published educational works are comparable to other forms of scholarship that are commonly used for promotion and tenure purposes (https://members.aamc.org/eweb/upload/MedEdPORTALEducationalScholarshipGuides.pdf). Education scholarship is now recognized as a valid domain that is rigorously peer-reviewed and is worthy as evidence of scholarship for decisions around promotion.

This chapter presents a broad introduction of the basic steps to conduct medical education research. The highlighted steps allow for the design of a robust research design taking into account some of the particular characteristics of an educational context, which can be very different from clinical science research.

Conceptual Frameworks

Conceptual frameworks represent ways of thinking about a problem or a study or ways of representing how complex things work the way they do [1]. These frameworks are critical in medical education research as they provide evidence that researchers have a thorough understanding of the field they are studying and help others to understand the theoretical rationale for the study. In addition, they contribute to programmatic scholarship in which researchers share common approaches and can build on each other's work [2].

Conceptual frameworks are based on theories, models, or evidence-based best practices and, as researcher Georges Bordage explains, are like lighthouses and magnifying lens: "Whereas the lighthouse illuminates certain parts of the ocean at any given time, other parts are left in the dark. A framework highlights or emphasizes different aspects of a problem or research question. Any one conceptual framework presents a partial view of reality. By contrast, they are also like magnifying glasses; each framework magnifies certain elements of a problem" [1].

For example, if a researcher were designing a method to teach intubation, a behaviorist approach would highlight skill-based practice and performance, a cognitivist approach would focus on developing mental models, and a social learning theory approach would emphasize learning through interaction between and among students and faculty. When considering frameworks, it is helpful to explore the range of options first as more than one may be relevant to the question or problem at hand. Thereafter, a researcher can decide which clarifies the situation best and use that framework to propose a study plan or solution. Specifically, the conceptual framework then "sets the stage" for presentation of the specific research question [3].

Research Question

The single most important component of a study is the research question [4]. In fact, the top reason given by reviewers for accepting manuscripts is that researchers addressed a timely and important question [5]. In proposing a research question, researchers can demonstrate that their work is relevant, advances the field forward, and addresses key practical or theoretical issues.

A research question should be suitable for examination and should be meaningful, clear, and relevant [6]. Refining the study question requires attention to a literature review and conceptual framework [7]. Beginning with a topic of interest, a medical education researcher progresses from broad and general questions to more precise and specific ones. The four key elements of a clear research question include the target population, the intervention or independent variable, the outcome or dependent variable, and the nature of the relationship between the variables. For example, a researcher may ask whether simulation training of intubation on a task trainer (intervention) results in higher rates (nature of the relationship between variables) of intubation success in clinical practice (outcome) among first year anesthesiology residents (target population). Alternatively, the researcher may consider the impact of two interventions on the same outcomes as in: Does simulation training of intubation on a task trainer (intervention 1) or video demonstration of intubation on a task trainer (intervention 2) result in higher rates (nature of the relationship between variables) of intubation success in clinical practice (outcome) among first year anesthesiology residents (target population)? The nature of the relationship is crucial in selecting optimal data analyses and drawing appropriate conclusions [5]. Therefore, it is important to note that the type and nature of the research question will determine whether a quantitative, qualitative, or mixed-methods approach is appropriate.

Once the research question has been identified, the next task is to decide on the study design. Will this be a retrospective review of data already gathered or is this an intervention from which change will be prospectively measured? Will there be a sufficient population to conduct a case–control study or will change for an entire group be measured? There are multiple decisions to be made, but these considerations fall into three main categories:

1. Who will be studied?
2. How will data be collected?
3. How will data be analyzed?

Study Population

The primary decision around the study population is in regard to whether this is a retrospective or prospective study. In a retrospective study, the researcher is somewhat limited in analyses based upon the available data. Still, such a study can provide useful information as a baseline or to set a standard for current practice. A prospective study, on the other hand, allows for more creativity in how the study is designed as well as in the collection and analysis of data. Based upon the number of available participants (residents, students, etc.) for a study, one can determine how long to collect data and how long to wait before an expected result. Power calculations provide necessary data to decide on sample sizes or the related power of studies based upon predetermined sample sizes, as in the case when one may be limited to the students in a particular training class. Many educational institutions offer free power analysis tools online to researchers who may not have these tools readily accessible otherwise.

Data Collection

The methods used for research vary depending on the research question(s). Qualitative research is used to capture meaning, to describe, or to understand the experiences and thoughts of participants in a particular setting [8]. It can also supplement quantitative data by explaining the results. Assessing faculty on a 1–5 scale on their teaching ability provides an overall rating but not why their teaching was effective or ineffective. Asking the rater to provide qualitative information about the teacher's strengths and weaknesses provides the "why." This methodology is best for answering a question such as "What residency learning experiences were most valuable to anesthesiology house staff?" or "How do academic faculty balance patient care, teaching, and research responsibilities?" The data that one collects is carefully reviewed and interpreted for common themes and trends (data reduction), both across and by subject, before the researcher extrapolates meaning from the data (data interpretation) [9]. One needs to understand that as data are analyzed, personal biases and beliefs may affect the interpretation. Good qualitative research acknowledges these potential biases and illustrates how they may be reflected in the data. Qualitative methods are becoming more common in educational research yet can be more challenging for a novice researcher.

Quantitative research is the more frequent method for scientific research in general. Through well-defined statements of hypotheses, methods, and findings, it seeks to eliminate any of the potential biases of a qualitative study and lend objectivity to the process [8]. Quantitative research requires careful planning at the beginning of a study to understand who or what is to be studied, how they or it will be assessed, and how will the data be analyzed, all in pursuit of answering your research question. Quantitative studies often are designed as a case–control design—such a design may have unique challenges in an education setting. It may be easier to design a pre- and post-intervention evaluation of the entire study group for your purposes. Data analysis normally requires some type of statistical testing, which can range from basic t-tests to sophisticated multivariate procedures. Depending on the researcher's skill set, partnering with a statistician may be indicated if plans require more sophisticated methods.

There are multiple ways to collect data to determine the effectiveness of a teaching intervention, including administrative data such as board scores or preceptor evaluations. From the participants' perspective, a survey or interviews, either one-on-one or in focus groups, may be indicated. Creating a personal survey, or evaluation tool, can be challenging. If there is a validated tool already available to measure the outcome, it should be used. It is always easier to use something that has already been tested for reliability and validity than to "invent" a new one. However, the fact is that in much of educational research, the settings are too context-specific to relate to broadly designed scales. If it is necessary to create a measurement tool "de novo," the most important thing to consider is proper wording of the questions and response choices. Item development is as much an art as a science and the best way to learn is to write down items and share them with colleagues for input. Dillman [10] is an excellent reference in guidance on writing questions, as is DeVellis [11] in the development of a scale. Regardless of a comfort level with potential survey questions, pretesting with a small group that is representative of the study population is essential. Only they can ensure that the items are interpreted in the intended fashion.

The most important step for research to develop a new outcome measure is to ensure the reliability and validity of data. Reliability refers to the ability of measures to provide reproducible data for meaningful interpretation [12]. In a test–retest situation, any change in score should be due to student behavior rather than a faulty measurement tool. Generally, a determination of reliability takes the form of some type of correlation function. If the assessment tool looks to measure how students answer the questions, a correlation analysis comparing, for example, a random two-halves of the test takers would provide one measure of reliability. If, on the other hand, the assessment is meant to be used as a tool for say, multiple preceptors to rate a student, we would be more interested in calculating some form of inter-rater reliability such as the kappa statistic. Here reliability refers to the ability of multiple individuals to use the same tool to measure a particular phenomenon. In all cases, there is no specific cutoff point to determine reliability, although a value of 0.90 or higher is desired.

A reliable tool measures something accurately over time. However, reliability does not ensure that the tool is measuring the *right* thing. Determining validity substantiates that a tool is measuring the intended construct(s). It provides data and evidence that support interpretation of scores [13]. This evidence is drawn from both theory and the collected data. There are many types of validity measures which can range from expert review of the survey items to statistical analyses of the inter-item correlations and overall structure of the survey tool. Efforts to determine reliability and validity might both require consultation with a statistician if these methods are not within the researcher's expertise.

Dissemination of Medical Education Research

There are several venues for presentation of data based upon the stage of completion. Consider first submitting preliminary results for a poster or oral presentation. Many academic medical centers or specific departments offer Education Research Day where preliminary results can be presented either orally or via poster. (If a department does not offer this opportunity, check with the affiliated medical school.) This opportunity initiates the process of organizing data for submission and can provide important feedback about research and any issues with presentation, such as clarity of the conceptual framework or how the results are represented, organization of the data, and relevance or applicability of the work. It can also provide an avenue for identifying parties who are interested in collaborating. In addition, presentation of the work can be extended to weekly or monthly departmental conferences or to regional, national, and international meetings that accept submissions. Education-focused organizations like International Association of Medical Science Educators (IAMSE) and the American Association of Medical Colleges (AAMC) have education conferences that might be interested in education research. The AAMC has the Group for Educational Affairs (GEA) that has national and regional groups. These groups hold annual meetings where research in medical education is presented both orally and via poster. Check the AAMC website (https://members.aamc.org/eweb/DynamicPage.aspx?webcode=MeetingHome) for meeting times, locations, and submission deadlines. Submission to these meetings is of value prior to completing a manuscript.

There are several educational venues where work can be disseminated, even during the process of completing research. The AAMC MedEdPORTAL is an excellent place for presenting research ideas. *iCollaborative*, one of three MedEdPORTAL sections, promotes the sharing of and collaboration on innovative educational ideas being developed and tested at member institutions. iCollaborative submissions differ from those in *Publications* in that they are not MedEdPORTAL peer-reviewed, they may not have yet been classroom tested, and they may not be fully functioning as a complete learning module. The purpose of *iCollaborative* is just to share ideas with the community.

A new teaching format, curriculum that has been taught or a new assessment tool, and preliminary results and/or feedback can be submitted through the MedEdPORTAL Publications section. MedEdPORTAL Publications serves as a clearinghouse of peer-reviewed health education tools. One must have stand-alone content, own all the materials, have classroom tested them, and provide privacy permission. The submissions are peer-reviewed by invited experts, cover the continuum of health education, and are open access, available to the general public internationally. Examples include teaching resources for faculty and advanced pain life support training materials [14]. The materials are recognized as scholarship and the formal citation and impact usage data from the site can be included in your educator portfolio.

Submissions to most journals require IRB approval or exemption from all institutions involved in the research, and this should be obtained prior to beginning research. Most education research can qualify for IRB exemption, especially if the results are anonymized. Each journal has its own requirements regarding the format of the presentation and each has different requirements for word length, category headings, numbers of figures and tables, format of the presentation (font, page number, margin size, etc.), and whether the verification of authorship, conflict of interest, and IRB paperwork are submitted with the original submission or only once it has been accepted for publication. Even negative studies can be published if they impact on what educators do in their daily work.

About Plagiarism

When writing up educational research, the same standards should be used as with any other scientific research. Any presentation of the research should appropriately acknowledge all relevant literature. For publication, all authors are held responsible and are required to sign a document indicating their contribution to the work.

Presenting Results

Prior to beginning research, it is helpful to identify a venue for presenting the work (meeting, journal publication) and the specific audience that will most likely find this work of interest and benefit from the results. Such an intervention helps to structure research and provide the framework for presentation of results. It is important to think of multiple potential short- and long-term conduits for results.

Results should be clear and easy to understand. The introduction should indicate the relevance of the work to the audience and the conceptual framework of the research, including how the research question is framed and resolved. The results section should only state the facts and the data. The results section should be organized either by theme or by research question and mirror the order presented in the introduction and in the other sections or could be presented based upon the type of data collected (quantitative versus qualitative). Use subsections within the results section if there are multiple themes. The results need to be consistent with the methodology. Tables and figures should only be used to present complex results or relationships between results. The text references the tables and figures but does not repeat all their results and simply describes and highlights key aspects. If submitting for publication, all the results should be presented and addressed.

The discussion should provide the reader with a context for the results and establish their relevance. It is where the results are interpreted as well as providing the implications of findings and the relationship of the results to other studies. Conclusions should be accurate and justified by results and follow from the research design, methods, and results. Also, identification and explanation of potential personal biases or influences on data analysis should be identified. Interpretation of results, limitations in research design, and future studies or plans should be laid out. Figure 15.1 highlights some key steps for any educational research project.

- Select an issue or topic of value to your department, facilitating buy-in from your department chair or division chief
- Do a literature search to identify what has been done and how you can add to the existing literature
- Develop a clear research question and consider your conceptual framework
- Collaborate with another educator in your department or in a similar department within or outside your institution. This will divide the work, likely increase your sample size and the diversity of your study population, enhance the research generalizability and may provide the impetus to stay on task and facilitate chances of publication.
- Identify a research mentor and other consultants and resources required to support you and the research you are engaged in
- Create a timeline and build in dedicated time to focus on the project
- Identify a realistic publication site and review their criteria in advance of starting your research

Fig. 15.1 Key steps for research in education

Foundation for Anesthesia Education and Research

Established in 1986, the mission of Foundation for Anesthesia Education and Research (FAER) is to facilitate continuous improvements in anesthesiology by supporting education, research, and scientific progress (www.faer.org). Grant proposals are reviewed, ranked, scored, and critiqued by the American Society of Anesthesiologists committee on research or the FAER education study section. As of 2013, research grants exceeding $20 million have been awarded to medical students, residents, and fellows in anesthesiology. In addition, in 2005, the Medical Student Anesthesia Research Fellowship Program was established to provide summer research opportunities. For anesthesiology residents beginning careers in academia and research, the FAER Resident Scholar Program provides a gateway to up-to-date knowledge in the specialty. More recently, a mentorship program has been added whereby noted academicians can share their expertise with trainees.

Conclusion

Beginning with the conceptual framework and research question, followed by careful consideration of the study design and population, a researcher can build a robust protocol and scholarship agenda. Recommendations for presentation and publication of scholarly activity include a systematic approach to study educational innovations and practice advances in the field and faculty career development in academic medicine.

References

1. Bordage G. Conceptual frameworks to illuminate and magnify. Med Educ. 2009;43(4):312–9.
2. Schwartz A, Pappas C, Bashook PG, et al. Conceptual frameworks in the study of duty hours changes in graduate medical education: a review. Acad Med. 2011;86(1):18–29.
3. McGaghie WC, Bordage G, Shea JS. Problem statement, conceptual framework, and research question. Acad Med. 2001;76(9):923–4.
4. Marks RG, Dawson-Saunders EK, Bailar JC, Dan BB, Verran JA. Interactions between statisticians and biomedical journal editors. Stat Med. 1988;7(10):1003–11.
5. Bordage G, Dawson B. Experimental study design and grant writing in eight steps and 28 questions. Med Educ. 2003;37(4):376–85.
6. Boet S, Sharma S, Goldman J, Reeves S. Review article: medical education research: an overview of methods. Can J Anaesth. 2012;59(2):159–70.
7. Beckman TJ, Cook DA. Developing scholarly projects in education: a primer for medical teachers. Med Teach. 2007;29(2–3):210–8.
8. Harwell MR. Research design in qualitative/quantitative/mixed methods. In: Conrad CF, Serlin RC, editors. The Sage handbook for research in education. 2nd ed. Los Angeles, CA: Sage; 2011. p. 147.
9. Miles MB, Huberman AM. Qualitative data analysis. 2nd ed. Los Angeles, CA: Sage; 1994.
10. Dillman DA. Mail and internet surveys. 2nd ed. New York, NY: Wiley; 2000.
11. DeVellis RF. Scale development: theory and applications. 3rd ed. Los Angeles, CA: Sage; 2012.
12. Downing SM. Reliability: on the reproducibility of assessment data. Med Educ. 2004;38: 1006–12.
13. Downing SM. Validity: on the meaningful interpretation of assessment data. Med Educ. 2003; 37:830–7.
14. Trescot A, Lollo L, Stogicza A. Advanced Pain Life Support (APLS) simulation training for interventional pain physicians. MedEdPORTAL; 2012. Available from: www.mededportal.org/publication/9240

Chapter 16
The Place of Global Education in Anesthesia

Angela Enright

Abbreviations

AAGBI	Association of Anaesthetists of Great Britain and Ireland
ABA	American Board of Anesthesiology
ASA	American Society of Anesthesiologists
ASA	Australian Society of Anaesthetists
CASIEF	Canadian Anesthesiologists' Society International Education Foundation
GAT	Group of Anaesthetists in Training
HIV	Human immunodeficiency virus
RCoA	Royal College of Anaesthetists
USA	United States of America
WEIGHT	Working Group on Ethics Guidelines for Global Health Training
WFSA	World Federation of Societies of Anaesthesiologists

Introduction

The world has changed markedly in recent decades and, with it, the world of medical education. This is a global environment and students require, and demand, a global view. Medical students are requesting programs that prepare them to work in the global health arena [1]. In many cases, the students are leading the demand and the faculty and medical schools are following.

Universities have developed Centers for Global Health [2–4] that assist faculty and students to engage, in very broad ways, in the greater world outside the home institutions and countries. No longer are students educated for practice in a local,

A. Enright (✉)
University of British Columbia, Royal Jubilee Hospital, Victoria, BC, Canada
e-mail: ape@telus.net

limited environment. They are interested in the world around them. They are philanthropic by nature. They want to see and experience health care in low-income settings. They are going to be "global health practitioners" [5]. By 2010, 37.5 % of American and Canadian medical schools had a global health component in their curriculum [6].

What Is Global Health?

Global health is defined as "service, training and research that address health problems disproportionately affecting resource-poor communities" [6]. These communities can exist in rich countries, e.g., the United States of America (USA) and Canada, as well as overseas. However, according to MacFarlane [1], global health is primarily defined by developed-country institutions in terms of these facilities working with developing countries. He says, "there is a danger that all this new energy for global health will result in it becoming an activity developed through the lens of rich countries, ostensibly for the benefit of poor countries, but without the key ingredients of a mutually agreed, collaborative endeavor." This attitude brings with it risks of accusations of paternalism and colonialism. A concerted effort is required to ensure that the needs and aspirations of all of those involved are addressed, that there is benefit to all participants, and that there is mutual understanding of, and agreement with, the goals of the programs.

Goals of Global Health Education

There are many goals for rotations in global health including exposure to different cultures and to different health systems, better understanding of public health challenges in low-income settings [5], exposure to tropical medicine [7], and improved understanding of the global burden of disease, inequalities, health and human rights [6]. These objectives are generally the same whether the learner is a medical student, resident or faculty member.

McKimm [8] describes the global health practitioner as someone who is clinically competent, who has the interpersonal skills to work in a multi-professional team, who uses resources judiciously, who can adapt to changing societal expectations, who contributes to medical scientific knowledge, and who can function effectively and flexibly in an ever-changing and unpredictable world, across cultures and under different social conditions. Participation in international health electives would be expected to provide exposure to, and experience in, many of these areas.

Our communities are changing and the need for cultural competence is very evident. 30 % of the population of the USA is made up of ethnic minorities [9]. Graduates need to be able to deal with patients from many different backgrounds and to understand the effects of varying cultures on health-care needs. Medical schools and residency training programs need to embed cultural training in their curricula. The Institute of Medicine in its treatise on health-care disparities states that, in the USA, racial and ethnic minorities experience lower-quality health care [10]. There is a need to promote global health while providing for local requirements.

Benefits of Global Health Electives to Residents

As medical students graduate and enter residency training, they continue their interest in global health [9, 11, 12]. There are many reports describing the setup, organization, and results of international health electives [6, 7, 13–15]. The themes are similar through every report.

The goals are the same as for the medical students but, because the residents are further advanced in their training, they bring more knowledge and skill to the projects and in return generally gain more benefits. Early adopters of international health electives for residents have been programs in family medicine, pediatrics, internal medicine, and emergency medicine. In 1998, 43 % of family medicine residencies in the USA offered international health electives [12]. Surgery has followed but there is little in the literature about anesthesia residents and global health electives.

Anesthesia residents in Canada and the USA have demonstrated significant interest in overseas work. Since 2006, about 46 residents have participated in the Rwanda project run by the Canadian Anesthesiologists' Society International Education Foundation (CAS IEF) and the American Society of Anesthesiologists (ASA) (Prof F. Carli, personal communication). Residents have also participated in activities organized by individual departments of anesthesia, e.g., University of California at San Francisco and Makerere University in Kampala, Uganda (Dr. G. Dubowitz, personal communication).

There is no formal statement about such electives and how they fit into residency training by the Royal College of Physicians and Surgeons of Canada [16]. The American Board of Anesthesiology (ABA) provides an application form for preapproval of nonaccredited electives [17]. The paucity of information from these two bodies is in marked contrast to the Royal College of Anaesthetists (RCoA) in the United Kingdom which has an explicit description of what the trainee should learn during a rotation in a low-income environment [18]. In addition, the Association of Anaesthetists of Great Britain and Ireland (AAGBI) has information and grants available for residents going abroad [19]. The Group of Anaesthetists in Training (GAT) has produced a very helpful booklet for those wishing to do any training outside their program including a section on electives in resource-poor environments [20]. In Australia and New Zealand, there is a formal link with the School of Medicine in Suva, Fiji, where anesthetic registrars can go to work and teach for up to 1 year. This is usually done at an advanced level of training. Some financial support is available from the Australian Society of Anaesthetists (ASA) (Dr. R. McDougall, personal communication).

The benefits of such rotations can be divided into three categories: (1) educational benefits, (2) skills, and (3) attitudes [12]. Educational benefits include increase in knowledge in many areas: alternative models of health care, public health issues, managing with few resources, effects of culture on health care, and advanced states of disease. Skills in diagnosis are enhanced by more reliance on history and physical examination and less on laboratory testing. Problem solving and language skills improve. Electives abroad often bring about a change in attitude and values, increase idealism, and foster interest in working in underserviced areas or with disadvantaged groups.

Students and residents who have done international electives have reported that they had improved skills and confidence, increased sensitivity to cost issues, decreased reliance on technology, and improved cross-cultural communication skills [9]. These are useful attributes to possess no matter where these residents or students subsequently practice.

Campbell describes a particular surgical mission organized by Operation Smile to celebrate its 25th anniversary [9]. Twenty-one plastic surgery residents received pre-trip preparation, then participated in various missions under the close supervision of mentors, and were then surveyed 1 year later. There was over 90 % response to the survey. One hundred percent of the respondents agreed that the mission had a positive impact on their lives and that it was a quality educational opportunity; 94.7 % said they achieved marked personal growth, that it was a valuable part of their training, and that they would take the opportunity to go on an international mission in the future if it was available.

Pre-mission Preparation

In the mission described above, the trainees were very well prepared but is that always the case? Tulane [13], Weill Cornell [6], Mayo Clinic [15], and Duke Universities [7] all describe the preparation they provide for their residents going abroad. Generally it involves some degree of orientation to the site and often it includes course work and seminars. Some insist on a review of the travel advisories from the Department of State to ensure that the region is safe. Most demand proof of immunization and a visit to a travel health clinic for information and advice on prevention and treatment of infectious diseases. It should be mandatory to purchase medical insurance that covers emergency evacuation if necessary.

Weill Cornell has developed a curriculum [6] with two main goals: (1) to provide a comprehensive overview of major thematic topics in global health and (2) to provide a mentored pathway for engaging with resource-poor communities both internationally and domestically. Five core competencies are defined for those taking a rotation in global health: (1) global burden of disease; (2) inequalities, health and human rights; (3) research- and evidence-based outcomes; (4) key stakeholders in global health; and (5) health systems and health-care delivery. This is a very comprehensive review of health care in its widest meaning and would be a good model for other universities and departments considering the development of international health electives for their students and residents.

There are some very practical programs available for anyone in anesthesia wishing to prepare for a mission abroad. The Department of Anaesthesia, Oxford University, in the United Kingdom, runs a 5-day "Anaesthesia in Developing Countries" course in Kampala, Uganda, to prepare anesthesiologists for work in a low-resource environment [21]. There are similar courses available in Australia "The Real World Anesthesia Course" [22] and in Canada and the USA "The Global Health Outreach Course" [23]. All of these courses have a similar theme, i.e., to expose the anesthesiologist to working conditions, different cultures, and the challenges of anesthesia in low-income countries. The courses accept small numbers of participants so the teacher-student ratio is very high. The instructors are uniquely experienced in working overseas in a variety of environments and are enthused about sharing their knowledge with the participants. The Global Health Outreach Course has been running in Canada since 2008 and approximately 40 anesthesia residents have participated (Dr. T. Coonan, personal communication). Feedback from all of these courses is very positive about how well the participants are prepared for their overseas experience.

Global Health Electives and Departments

What benefits do departments of anesthesia receive from facilitating participation in global health electives by their residents and faculty? In the USA, there is a sense that residents preferentially select programs that offer these types of electives [7, 15]. Departments benefit from the increased confidence and skills of their trainees. They demonstrate improved cross-cultural communication [9] and, as a result, deal more effectively with patients. They may be more aware of cost issues. International health electives have the potential to be incorporated into residency training programs. Ninety-two percent of surgical residents surveyed by the American College of Surgeons [9] were interested in such rotations; 82 % of those surveyed said they would prioritize them over other electives. There is a strong appeal to the reasons why people went into medicine in the first place. Residents who pursue overseas electives often have the opportunity to teach and that also appeals to them. They have a sense of contributing something valuable.

Challenges to International Electives

There are many obstacles to overcome for both departments and individuals in pursuing international electives. For the participant, it is often difficult to adjust to a new culture on arrival and to readjust to the home culture on return [15]. Learning to work without the usual equipment, tools, and supports can be difficult.

The severity of the illnesses and conditions encountered can be overwhelming. Death on a frequent basis can be very discouraging. Even the numbers of patients requiring care can be overpowering.

Residents can also be concerned for their personal welfare and safety. There is increased risk of infectious illness—blood-borne such as human immunodeficiency virus (HIV), water- or food-borne such as diarrhea, and vector-borne such as malaria [7]. General safety can also be a concern depending on location and political stability.

There are other factors that worry residents such as salary continuance, costs of travel, separation from family, and accommodation requirements. Many worry about their ability to cope in challenging environments. They need reassurance that their rotation will receive academic approval.

For the departments, there are concerns for the safety and well-being of the resident. It is more reassuring to have trainees going to centers where the department has strong links on an ongoing basis. Finding suitable host programs can be difficult. Departments must be reassured that there is appropriate supervision of trainees. This could be by local host faculty or by visiting teachers. There has to be proper administrative and financial support of the program [15]. In spite of all these challenges, international rotations are popular and well supported [11].

Host Departments and Faculty

MacFarlane says that "academic institutions have an opportunity and responsibility to ensure that global health is inclusive and world-wide" [1]. Inclusive should mean that host institutions and faculty ought to benefit from the process. It should be beneficial for all participants not just those visiting from a high-income country. Yet, in all of the literature reviewed, there is very little mention of reciprocity for visits and support for local faculty. Chiller suggests that, where feasible, student exchanges should go both ways and that salaries of supervising faculty physicians be supplemented [13]. He also suggests that, if there is no medical school, a Continuing Medical Education fund be set up for paraprofessionals.

One of the aims of educating physicians in global health is to help them understand the difficulties of practicing medicine in a low-income setting. There are immense shortages not only of anesthesiologists [24, 25] but of all trained anesthesia providers [26, 27]. There are programs in several African countries where ongoing relationships have developed between mentor programs in North America and a local university or hospital. One such program is in Rwanda with a very mutually beneficial relationship between the Canadian Anesthesiologists' Society International Education Foundation, the American Society of Anesthesiologists, and the National University of Rwanda. Volunteer faculty go to Rwanda to teach in the residency training program. These faculty members are frequently accompanied by residents in training. Rwandan residents go to Canada for part of their training. Local faculty, including the Residency Program Director, have spent time in Canadian departments increasing their knowledge of administration and program development. Small joint research projects have been funded, published, and presented in tandem. In general it is a mutually beneficial arrangement [28].

Another such project is in place at Makerere University in Kampala, Uganda, where several universities participate [29]. The University of California at San Francisco and the University of British Columbia in Vancouver both work with the Department of Anesthesia in Kampala to train anesthesia residents. Faculty and residents from both go to Kampala and faculty and residents from Kampala spend time in Vancouver and San Francisco. Long-term relationships have been established and flourish.

McMaster University in Hamilton, Ontario has a long established relationship with Mbarara University in Southern Uganda. Faculty members and residents are exchanged between both universities. McMaster utilizes the adage "Come and see; go and tell" (Dr. A. Dauphin, personal communication). It is a mutually beneficial relationship for both groups.

It is vital that relationships between rich and poor departments not contribute to the "brain-drain." Of course, people will move for a variety of reasons but appropriate support from external departments could, and should, encourage local faculty to stay and further develop their own departments. Support for the development and sustenance of training programs, fostering of an academic environment by provision of education materials, sharing of expertise in developing a research agenda, assistance with writing, publications and presentations could all be part of a two-way program. Introducing safety practices that are affordable such as the use of the Surgical Safety Checklist could reduce anesthetic and surgical morbidity and mortality [30].

Departments of anesthesia sending residents to train in departments with few resources could also assist with the development of curricula [31]. Importing a curriculum from abroad is not often appropriate to the location or circumstances. But working with local faculty to ensure that there is a balance between what is essential in the local environment and an introduction to new anesthetic techniques and equipment is important in encouraging further development within departments. Local faculty and residents read of and hear about new approaches, e.g., ultrasound-guided regional anesthesia, and, even if they do not have an ultrasound available, they want to know and understand the principles.

Another no-cost way of assisting departments is to share with them new approaches to teaching. Many still use only traditional didactic teaching so coaching them to use small group sessions, problem-based learning, scenario teaching, and resident presentations can improve learning and make classroom sessions more interesting. The World Federation of Societies of Anaesthesiologists (WFSA) pioneered a Teach the Teachers training program in anesthesia [32]. It has now had about 80 participants from 21 European countries and has begun in Latin America with 40 anesthesiologists from 10 countries. It is now preparing to launch in Africa (Dr. W. Morriss, personal communication). Introducing task trainers and simulation models, team training, and crisis management opens up a whole new world of learning.

The Role of Ethics in Global Education

Introducing faculty and residents to issues in global anesthesia provides an opportunity to review ethical issues. There is a great need for ethical guidelines for medical staff and trainees traveling abroad for educational experiences [33]. The Working Group on Ethics Guidelines for Global Health Training (WEIGHT) published a set of guidelines in 2010. They include the roles and responsibilities of the sending and host institutions, the trainees, and the sponsors [34]. It is important that all parties benefit from the experience yet little is known of the effects on the host institution, host faculty or trainees. The guidelines emphasize the need for clear documentation and understanding from both sides. At a minimum they should be reviewed with each person participating in a global health experience. On returning from a trip, each resident should submit a report which would include a comment on any ethical issues encountered and whether or not preparation was adequate. Faculty from sending and host institutions should also review and update the ethical guidelines on a regular basis.

De Camp et al. devised an ethics curriculum for study before trainees go abroad [33]. It consists of ten case studies which have been developed from actual experiences of trainees [35]. Each vignette illustrates an important ethical question that a trainee might encounter. There is feedback on each answer and important ethical points are illustrated. The curriculum addresses three areas—trainee behavior, context of short-term programs, and research. A survey of people using this curriculum-website revealed that, of those who had been abroad previously, only 31 % had had ethics training related to short-term work; 34 % said this would be their only ethics training; 24 % reported that their training program had required them to take the curriculum; more than 70 % agreed that the cases gave them a structure for dealing with ethical questions.

This is not the only curriculum available. The University of British Columbia has an excellent online ethics forum which would be very helpful for trainees planning an educational trip overseas [36]. The cases are not necessarily related to medicine, but there are many themes that resonate and would be useful to consider prior to a planned overseas experience.

Conclusions

Overall it appears that encouraging residents to participate in global health electives is of benefit not only to the resident but also to the training program and possibly to the patients it serves. The resulting advantages can include a better global perspective on health care, awareness of the health needs of large segments of the world's population, an appreciation of alternative health-care models, and improved cross-cultural communication. There are risks involved in sending trainees abroad and these must be recognized and trainees prepared for them. Significant thought must be given to the needs of the host program. If the participating programs work and plan together toward shared goals, then these international programs can be of mutual benefit to all.

References

1. MacFarlane SB, Jacobs M, Kaaya EE. In the name of global health: trends in academic institutions. J Public Health Policy. 2008;29:383–401.
2. University of British Columbia Global Health. Available at https://globalhealth.med.ubc.ca. Accessed 26 April 2013.
3. Yale Global Health initiative. Available at https://ghi.yale.edu. Accessed 26 April 2013.
4. Duke Global Health Institute. Available at https://globalhealth.duke.edu. Accessed 26 April 2013.
5. Coupet S. International health electives: strengthening graduate medical education. J Am Osteopath Assoc. 2012;112:800–4.
6. Francis ER, Goodsmith N, Michelow M, et al. The global health curriculum of Weill Cornell Medical College: how one school developed a global health program. Acad Med. 2012;87:1296–302.
7. Miller WC, Corey GR, Lallinger GJ, Durack DT. International health and internal medicine residency training: The Duke University experience. Am J Med. 1995;99:291–7.
8. McKimm J, McLean M. Developing a global health practitioner: time to act? Med Teach. 2011;33:626–31.
9. Campbell A, Sullivan M, Sherman R, Magee WP. The medical mission and modern cultural competency training. J Am Coll Surg. 2011;212:121–9.
10. Institute of Medicine, National Academy of Sciences. Unequal treatment: confronting racial and ethnic health disparities in health care. Washington, DC: Institute of Medicine; 2002. Available at http://www.iom.edu/reports/2002/unequal-treatment-confronting-racial-and-ethnic-health-disparities-in-health-care.aspx. Accessed 21 April 2013.
11. Powell AC, Casey K, Liewehr DJ, et al. Results of a national survey of surgical resident interest in international experiences, electives and volunteerism. J Am Coll Surg. 2009;208:304–12.
12. Thompson MJ, Huntingdon MK, Hunt DD, et al. Educational effects of international health electives on US and Canadian medical students and residents: a literature review. Acad Med. 2003;78:342–7.
13. Chiller TM, De Mieri P, Cohen I. International health training: the Tulane experience. Infect Dis Clin North Am. 1995;9(2):439–43.
14. Gupta AR, Wells CK, Horwitz RI, et al. The international health program: the fifteen-year experience with Yale University's Internal Medicine Residency program. Am J Trop Med Hyg. 1999;61:1019–23.
15. Sawatsky AP, Rosenman DJ, Merry SP, McDonald FS. Eight years of the Mayo International Health program: what an elective adds to resident education. Mayo Clin Proc. 2010;85:734–41.
16. Royal College of Physicians and Surgeons of Canada. Available at http://rcpsc.medical.org/residency/certification/training/anesthesiology_e.pdf. Accessed 1 May 2013.
17. The American Board of Anesthesiology. Available at www.theaba.org/Training_Away_Checklist.pdf. Accessed 1 May 2013.
18. The Royal College of Anaesthetists. Annex D: higher level training in anaesthetics. p. 48. Available at www.rcoa.ac.uk. Accessed 1 May 2013.
19. The Association of Anaesthetists of Great Britain and Ireland. Available at www.aagbi.org/international. Accessed 1 May 2013.
20. The Association of Anaesthetists of Great Britain and Ireland. Organising a year abroad. Available at www.aagbi.org/sites/default/files/organising_year_abroad09.pdf. Accessed 1 May 2013.

21. Anaesthesia in developing countries. Available at http://www.nda.ox.ac.uk/courses/anaesthesiaHealth-in-developing-countries. Accessed 27 April 2013.
22. The Real World Anesthesia Course. Available at http://asa.org.au/events/future_events/detail/index_html?content_id=162706. Accessed 27 April 2013.
23. The Global Health Outreach Course. Available at http://anesthesia.medicine.dal.ca/global-health-outreach-course.php. Accessed 27 April 2013.
24. Dubowitz G, Detlefs S, McQueen KA. Global anesthesia work force crisis: a preliminary survey revealing shortages contributing to undesirable outcomes and unsafe practices. World J Surg. 2010;34:438–44.
25. Linden AF, Sekidde FS, Galukande M, et al. Challenges of surgery in developing countries: a survey of surgical and anesthesia capacity in Uganda's public hospitals. World J Surg. 2012;36:1056–65.
26. Enright AC. Review article: safety aspects of anesthesia in under-resourced locations. Can J Anaesth. 2013;60:152–8.
27. Spiegel DA, Choo S, Cherian M, et al. Quantifying surgical and anesthetic availability at primary care facilities in Mongolia. World J Surg. 2011;35:272–9.
28. Twagirumugabe T, Carli F. Rwandan anesthesia residency program: a model for north-south educational partnership. Int Anesthesiol Clin. 2010;48(2):71–8.
29. Lipnick M, Mijumbi C, Dubowitz G, et al. Surgery and anesthesia capacity building in resource-poor settings: description of an ongoing academic partnership in Uganda. World J Surg. 2013;37:488–97.
30. Haynes AB, Weiser TG, Berry WR, et al. A surgical safety checklist to reduce morbidity and mortality in a global population. N Engl J Med. 2009;360:461–9.
31. Dubowitz G, Evans FM. Developing a curriculum for anesthesia training in low- and middle-income countries. Best Pract Res Clin Anaesthesiol. 2012;26(1):17–21.
32. World Federation of Societies of Anaesthesiologists. Education committee report 2008–2012. Available at www.anaesthesiologists.org/document-files/Education%202008-12.pdf. Accessed 10 May 2013.
33. DeCamp M, Rodriguez J, Hecht S, et al. An ethics curriculum for short-term global health trainees. Global Health. 2013,9:5. Available at http://www.globalizationandhealth.com/content/9/1/5. Accessed 10 May.
34. Crump JA, Sugarman J. and the Working Group on Ethics Guidelines for Global Health Training (WEIGHT). Global health training: ethics and best practice guidelines for training experiences in global health. Am J Trop Med Hyg. 2010;83:1178–82.
35. Ethical challenges in global health training. Available at http://ethicsandglobalhealth.org. Accessed 11 May 2013.
36. The ethics of international engagement and service-learning. Available at http://ethicsofisl.ubc.ca/. Accessed 11 May 2013.

Chapter 17
Community Outreach

Jordan Brand and Clifford Gevirtz

Introduction

Anesthesiology today is a technology-intensive specialty with an increasing spectrum of subspecialties ranging from perioperative patient care to pain management, critical care, and palliative care. Anesthesiologists can play a decisive role in patient management throughout the entire inpatient, ambulatory, and office experience. While we talk of newer and safer drugs, better drug delivery systems, and formulation of optimal management plans in terms of better perioperative management of vital functions and critical care, we tend to lose sight of the fact that the general population understands little of these developments. The problems of image and status of the anesthesiologists in the eyes of the medical and lay communities are certainly not new. Indeed we have been called the Rodney Dangerfield of medical specialties because of this low profile.

With the approach of the Accountable Care Act, the shifting healthcare environment, and continued advancement in anesthesiology, the patients and general public need to be educated about our role in their care and the benefits that we provide. We should highlight anesthesiology as a separate medical discipline in audiovisual as well as print and social media.

J. Brand, M.D. (✉)
Department of Anesthesiology, San Francisco VA Medical Center, University of California, 4150 Clement Street, San Francisco, CA 94121, USA
e-mail: jbrandmd@gmail.com

C. Gevirtz, M.D., M.P.H.
LSU Health Sciences Center, New Orleans, LA, USA
e-mail: cliffgevirtzmd@yahoo.com

Community Outreach Opportunities

Much of the training of anesthesiologists takes place in the operating room (OR), intensive care unit (ICU), pain clinic, and other direct-patient-care settings. However, there is an increasing trend towards involving residents and fellows in community outreach activities. Community outreach is a broad category that may include the following activities:

1. Free medical care (local or international)
2. Other interventions designed to increase access to care
3. Education of the public
4. Direct charitable activities

Taking part in such endeavors may lead to several benefits for trainees and practitioners: they develop greater awareness of the scope of the healthcare system, both nationally and globally, and an enhanced appreciation for the way income and socioeconomic inequalities affect the provision of care. In addition, by working in settings far afield from their comfort zones, anesthesiologists in training are forced to cultivate greater flexibility and improved interpersonal and communication skills.

Among many departments of anesthesiology that have developed major community outreach programs are Stanford University and Vanderbilt University to name just two. Tangible local outreach endeavors at Stanford include transport programs (Neonatal Critical Care Transport, Adult Critical Care Transport) that were developed to permit transportation of critical patients from institutions with inadequate facilities to Stanford hospitals. Additionally, a medical acupuncture division has been developed to provide alternative, yet effective therapies to patients with chronic pain and other conditions. Globally, many faculty have participated in medical volunteer efforts in disadvantaged countries of the world. Faculty and residents have also been involved in helping improve the health and well-being of endangered and exotic animal species. One of the most visible outreach initiatives at Vanderbilt is the Vanderbilt International Anesthesia program that allows faculty, staff, and trainees of the anesthesia department to extend clinical care to many underserved areas around the world through the provision of grants and awards of excellence to leaders and mentors.

The benefits of community outreach are not limited to individual participants. While they serve critical roles in the healthcare system, anesthesiologists are among the least-familiar specialists to the public. Indeed, up to 35 % of patients in some studies are unaware that anesthesiologists are even physicians [1]. Adding a further difficulty, when they do appear in the popular media, especially as portrayed by the film industry, anesthesiologists are frequently depicted as uninvolved, uncommitted to patient care, poorly educated, addicted to alcohol or drugs, or worse. Because the anesthesiologist is an "obligate" and not "voluntary" caregiver for most patients, little research is generally devoted to anesthesia by all but the most-educated healthcare consumers, making such misunderstandings possible. For such a specialty, therefore, it is of great importance to take advantage of any opportunity to present a good face to the public as well as to broaden understanding of anesthesiologists' role in perioperative care. Community outreach in anesthesia education thus serves a dual purpose: it benefits trainees by exposing them to a wider range of clinical and social situations, and it serves to improve the standing of the specialty in society as a whole.

Free Care and Improving Access to Care

The most traditional approach to community outreach in medicine is the provision of low- or no-cost medical care via a "free resident clinic." While this approach works well for primary-care specialties (and even some more specialized ones), anesthesiologists rarely practice in a vacuum and are not as familiar with the clinic environment, making such an arrangement more difficult. In some academic centers, residency training may involve participation in an internal medical clinic performing medical evaluation for patients prior to surgery. Such an arrangement carries an added benefit in that the anesthesia resident works alongside an internal medicine resident and thus gleans experience from yet another point of view and training.

But anesthesiologists are frequently able to provide free care in other ways, such as medical missions and charitable care for surgical patients. Because anesthesiologists cannot easily deliver care alone, such efforts require coordination with surgeons and other medical professionals, and while this can present some difficulties, it can also lead to deeper working relationships and a greater understanding between specialties.

Medical Missions

Numerous anesthesiology training programs offer the opportunity to participate in medical missions, an important intervention designed to increase access to care. Residents travel and work alongside anesthesia attendings, nurses, and other physicians to provide care for those in other countries who would not otherwise have access to it as well as teach new techniques to local practitioners. Numerous such teams make planned trips every year to developing countries and frequently respond to emergency situations such as the 2010 earthquake in Haiti [2]. Such missions provide much-needed medical care and also give trainees a broader perspective on global health and the spectrum of disease found worldwide (Figs. 17.1, 17.2, 17.3, and 17.4). In some resource-poor settings, anesthesiologists may have to bring their own supplies and alter techniques due to on-the-ground limitations. Trainees and even their leaders are forced to develop new skills in planning and flexibility. For instance, when advanced recovery-room care is not available, many procedures that would otherwise be better performed under general anesthesia must be completed with local or regional techniques and minimal or no sedation.

Over the past decade a relationship between the Icahn School of Medicine at Mount Sinai and a third world hospital in Honduras has been established. During annual surgical missions in this time, learning with each undertaking and

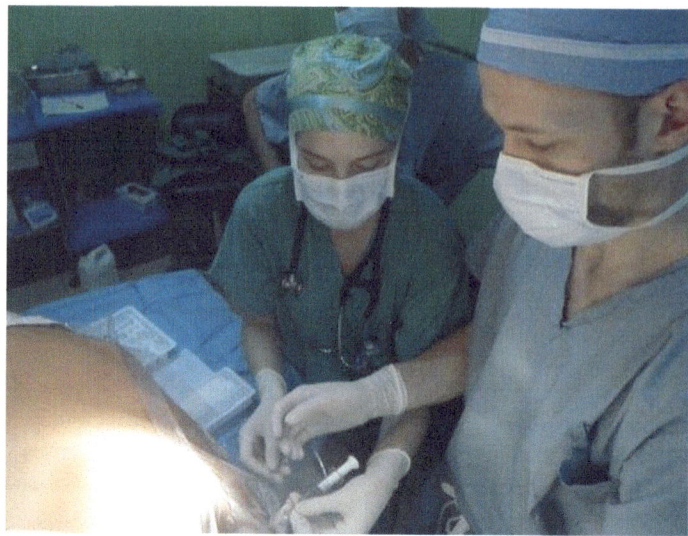

Fig. 17.1 An anesthesia resident and attending place an epidural catheter during a medical mission in Honduras. Photo courtesy of Ram Roth, M.D.

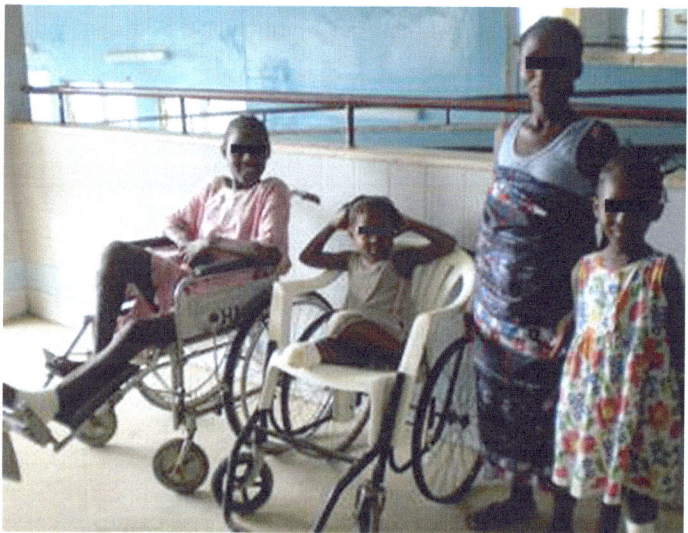

Fig. 17.2 Liberian children from the ward

adjustments had to be made. Three areas in particular were indentified that may help others in providing missions [3]:

1. An intensive medical student and global health curriculum was developed with major input from students. On average 10 students participated in each mission,

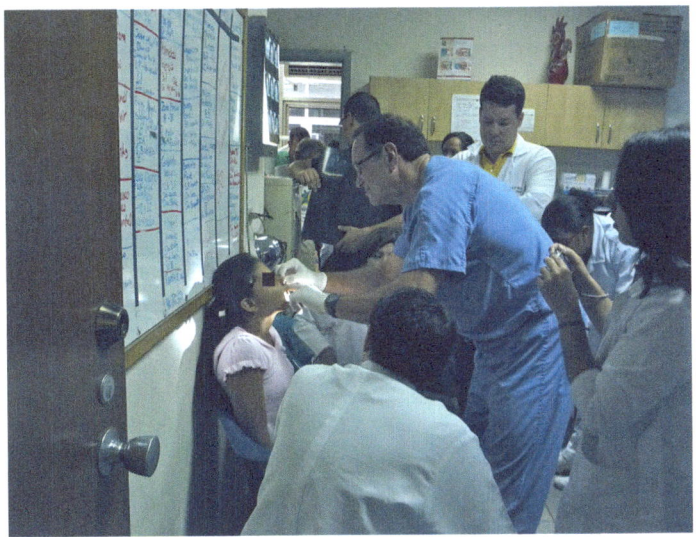

Fig. 17.3 Patients being screened by surgeons and staff in Honduras

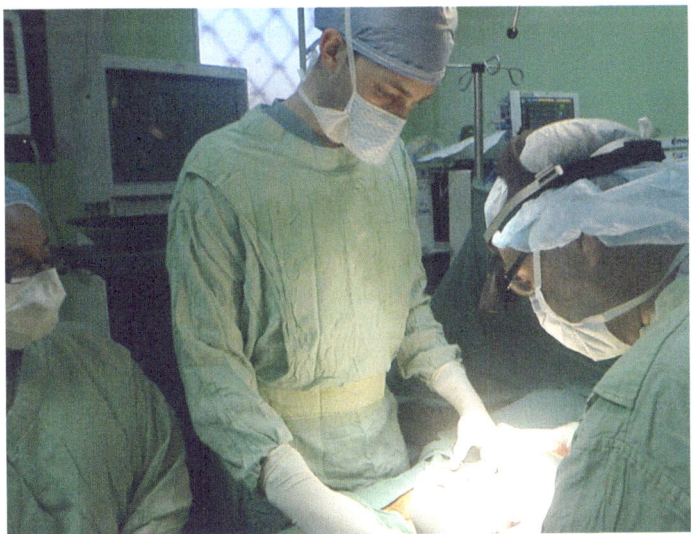

Fig. 17.4 Operating in a Honduran hospital. Note fewer instruments and light. Photo courtesy of Dr. Roth

alongside 3 resident and 3 attending anesthesiologists. The students promoted the relationship with the hospital, and overlapping of second and fourth year students provided continuity of care. Students gained perspective on patient care in resource-poor settings and also assumed critical roles in educating local healthcare providers and in organization as well as follow-up care.

2. Successful resuscitation of a witnessed cardiac arrest in a postsurgical patient emphasized the lack of available equipment and even the concept of a resuscitative team. Algorithms, drills, and a code box became a standard of care to help remedy these deficits and empower the local staff.
3. Missions last only 1–2 weeks usually and postoperative follow-up is often difficult relying on cell phone contact from the United States. Surveys made over several years indicated that short-term (1 month) contact yielded better results than long term (1 year) (62–8 %). Quick turnover in cell phone numbers in poor countries probably also contributed to the poor response at a later date. Repeated calling at different times of the day as well as better preoperative patient education, especially in ensuring current phone and family contact information, was clearly essential. Maintaining contact with local staff allowed improved follow-up information and retained good will.

International Scholar Programs

Both the New York State Society of Anesthesiologists and, to the lesser extent, the American Society of Anesthesiologists (ASA) have developed programs to help anesthesiologists from underdeveloped countries to come to national meetings to gain insight into what is being done in the United States and to gauge what they can reasonably translate back to care in their own countries.

Scholars receive different financial awards, determined by their application, ranging from free registration to shared hotel accommodation and, if funding allows, some contribution towards transportation costs. In addition, technical exhibitors and publishing firms often donate equipment and books rather than transporting the material back to warehouses at the end of a trade show. Scholars often present posters, a process that often ensures some financial support from their home institutions or even governments. Funding for such programs comes from private donations, sometimes set up through tax-exempt organization.

Observerships

Many departments allow observerships for anesthesiologists from other countries to permit these individuals to gain an insight into anesthetic care in the United States. These programs may last for 1–4 weeks or even longer. In most institutions, hands-on experience by the visitor is not permitted. Moreover, application for the programs may be difficult, requiring completion of extensive health questionnaires among many other forms. In departments that have access to a simulation lab, the process is clearly much simpler.

Systems-Based Practice

In addition to the needs of patients abroad, many individuals in developed countries may still fall through the cracks of the medical system and therefore require charitable care. "Systems-based practice," which refers to "awareness of and responsiveness to the larger context and system of health care and the ability to effectively call on system resources to provide care that is of optimal value," is one of the core competencies of the Accreditation Council for Graduate Medical Education (ACGME) [4]. This competency includes an understanding of the costs and economic issues that impact the delivery of healthcare. Unfortunately, many residents feel insulated from this issue [5]. Any opportunity to prompt discussion on how patients pay (or cannot pay) for their care is a step towards this goal. Likewise, while cost issues are unlikely to have a large effect on intraoperative care at an academic institution, they may impact perioperative care, such as choice of pain medications and opportunities for rehabilitation and follow-up management. To be truly effective as an educational tool, though, participation in charity care and medical missions must be a jumping-off point for further discussion, not the only step.

Lack of funds is not the only obstacle to obtaining care for many patients. Another example of an impediment that can be overcome with some effort is the language barrier. Over 8 % of Americans in some surveys have limited English proficiency, and this rate may be substantially higher in certain parts of the country. Patients with limited English skills are at risk for misdiagnoses and may be less likely to pursue appropriate follow-up care [6]. While interpreters are available at most academic medical centers, residents are rarely specifically trained in their effective use. Some direct education of residents in the appropriate usage of interpreters is helpful. Additionally, as many residents speak foreign languages fluently, it may be possible to match up patients with residents that share their languages to care for them in preoperative, operating room (OR), and postoperative settings. Such an intervention would likely take little additional effort and can increase not just the clarity of patient-doctor communication but build camaraderie between patients and caregivers.

Public Education

Just as anesthesiology residency incorporates aspects of clinical care and didactic education, community outreach is not limited to clinical care; it can also take the form of education of the nonmedical public. Every year, numerous departments of anesthesiology welcome high school and college students who have an interest in medicine in general and sometimes in anesthesia specifically. These students participate in didactic lectures, observe clinical care in and out of the OR, and often have the opportunity to take part in other activities such as medical simulation. In some cases, students may be able to follow patients longitudinally and gain a

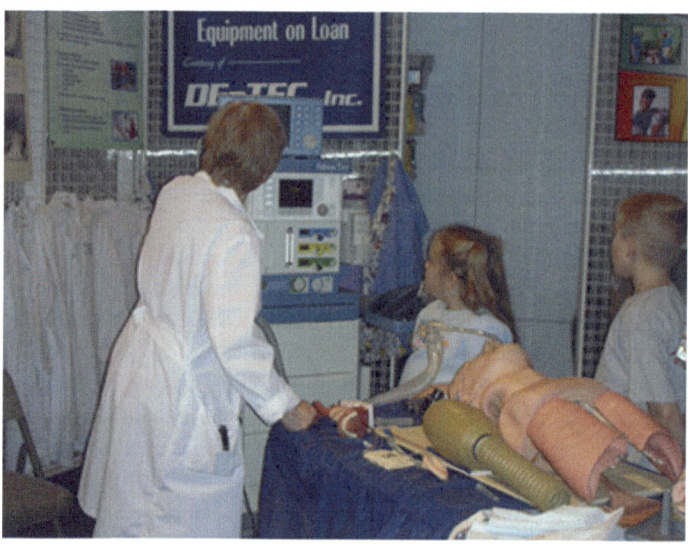

Fig. 17.5 Members of the New York State Society of Anesthesiologists at the annual New York State (NYS) Fair. Photos courtesy of the New York State Society of Anesthesiologists (NYSSA)

better understanding of their overall course through the perioperative period. Again, there is a dual benefit here: the students gain rich educational opportunities and have an all-too-rare chance to experience medicine firsthand before committing to premedical studies; residents are able to polish their educational and leadership skills. If trainees aspire to careers in academics, such an experience enables them to test the waters in a way that is not always available during residency. These programs comply with the medical dictum that the best way to learn something is to teach it.

Students are not the only ones this type of outreach may involve: some schools have started "mini-medical schools" that offer lectures directed at the nonmedical public. While few departments of anesthesiology have so far undertaken this course, there is no reason to leave anesthesia out of such a curriculum. Additionally, on a more populist level, groups such as the New York State Society of Anesthesiologists have created exhibits at state fairs and other public events to demonstrate anesthesia practice and answer people's questions about the specialty [7]. Such events are a good way not just to increase public awareness but also for trainees to gain a sense of shared mission and to improve interpersonal and communication skills (Figs. 17.5, 17.6, 17.7, and 17.8).

One way to educate the public about anesthesiology is to bring the outside world into the medical sphere; another is to produce work that places anesthesia and anesthesiologists in the public sphere. A handful of anesthesiologists have written books, both fiction and nonfiction, that cast anesthesiologists as their protagonists [8, 9]. Others have created books that are more explicitly designed to educate the public about the importance of anesthesiology [10]. Residents have rarely taken a leading

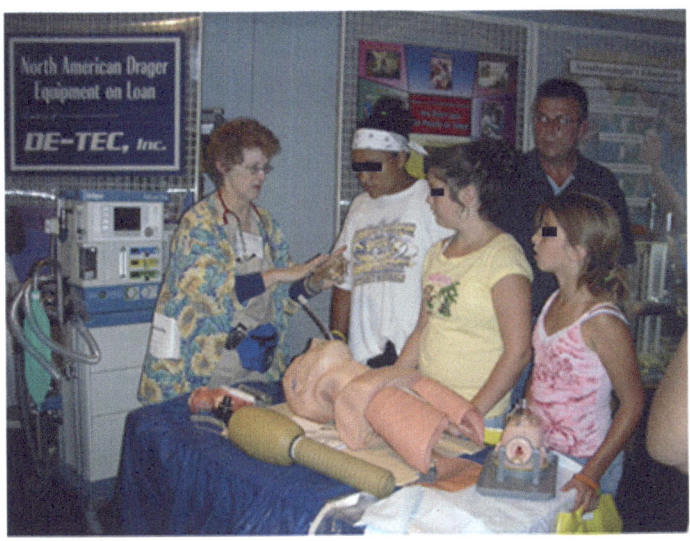

Fig. 17.6 Members of the New York State Society of Anesthesiologists at the annual NYS Fair. Photos courtesy of the NYSSA

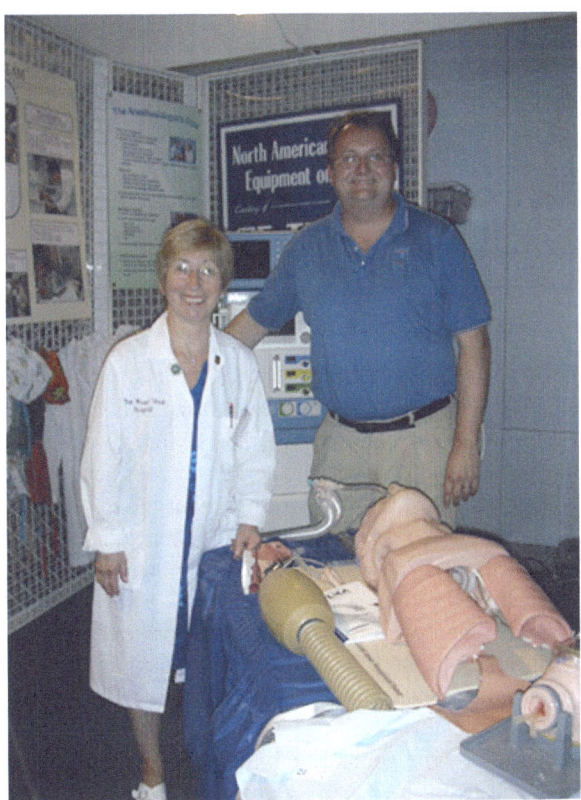

Fig. 17.7 Members of the New York State Society of Anesthesiologists at the annual NYS Fair. Photos courtesy of the NYSSA

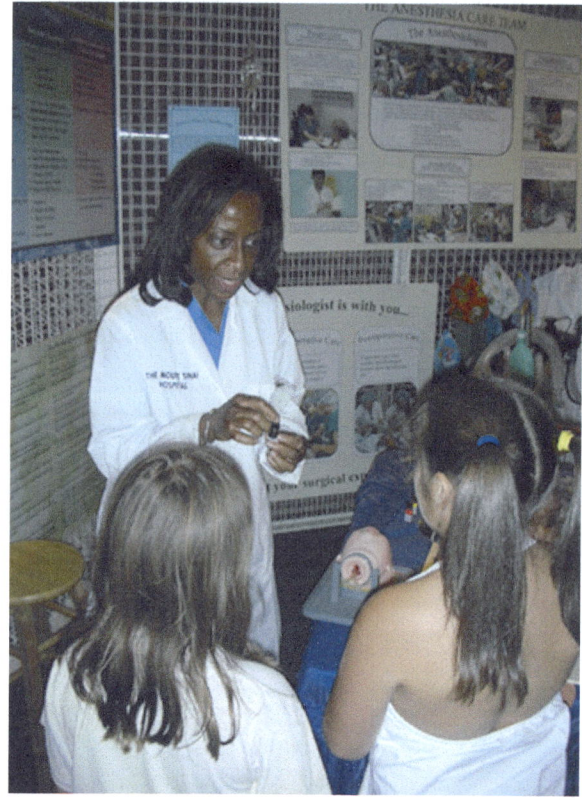

Fig. 17.8 Members of the New York State Society of Anesthesiologists at the annual NYS Fair. Photos courtesy of the NYSSA

role in these endeavors, but transforming the experience of medical training into a narrative can often be therapeutic and improve the quality of education. By learning narrative techniques, residents can enhance their ability to efficiently obtain and process patient histories as well as gain a greater sense of resiliency and empathy [11]. Therefore, there is reason to think that writing about the experience of residency training—in a realistic or unrealistic way—would be beneficial for the authors. Also likely to gain are readers who may be exposed to the rare sight of anesthesiologists stepping out from behind the ether screen.

While not generally regarded as "the public," other professionals may be less sure of the role of the anesthesiologist. Considerable advantage is obtained when surgeons and others, including nurses and administrators, are part of a multidisciplinary conference that helps other specialists gain insight into the role of the anesthesiologist. Such programs, spurred by the general findings of Joint Commission reviews that the majority of medical errors are due to lack of communication, are rapidly gaining momentum under the hubris of "TeamSTEPPS, Team Strategies to Enhance

Performance and Patient Safety Teamstepps.ahrq.gov." Educating the physicians or surgeons regarding our discipline has the added advantage of improving the knowledge that the patients get from them regarding our role in patient management.

Electronic, Print, and Blogs

The electronic and print media has a tremendous potential to educate the general population, but this potential has always been underutilized. By tapping into social and print media, there is a tremendous potential to educate the general population. When patients have prior knowledge through audiovisual or print media about anesthesiology, they may have expanded options to inquire and choose their anesthesiologist so that a less medically trained person (e.g., certified registered nurse anesthetist, CRNA) may not be the only provider of anesthesiology services.

To help educate and inform prospective patients and the public at large, the ASA has launched LifelinetoModernMedicine.com, the most comprehensive online resource on anesthesia care.

"Health care advancements and treatment options continue to expand rapidly, made possible by the anesthesiologists who oversee an estimated 40 million anesthetics administered in the U.S. each year," said Roger A. Moore, M.D., president of the American Society of Anesthesiologists (ASA). "Given the complexity of today's surgical procedures and the central role anesthesia plays in making those procedures possible, the ASA has launched this Web site with the aim that all patients become informed and educated about their care."

The general public and prospective patients will have access to various anesthesia-related resources and tools on LifelinetoModernMedicine.com, including:

- The Anesthesia & Me(C) checklist, a potentially lifesaving form that the ASA recommends people print, fill out, and keep in their wallets in case of surgery. The checklist details a person's medical history, current medications, allergies, and additional items necessary for proper anesthesia care.
- Information on the different types of anesthesia and the risks associated with each.
- Details about what to expect before and after surgery.
- Information on relevant medical specialties, including obstetrics, pediatrics, geriatric medicine, and acute, chronic, and cancer pain medicine.
- Real-life patient stories.

"Although millions of operations are performed each year, surgery is a big decision for every patient," said Moore. "LifelinetoModernMedicine.com gives patients a wealth of information so they can be well-informed about their options."

The ASA publishes a press kit each year, which can be utilized to obtain coverage in local and national media outlets.

The Hill is a congressional newspaper that publishes daily when the Congress is in session. This blog discusses all the issues of the day, especially as regards health matters. It represents a means to educate politicians regarding medical topics through a comment section.

The Anesthesiologist in Political Life

The future of anesthesia practice is being shaped by several external factors including scope of practice challenges by nonphysicians, declining levels of reimbursements, and changes in resident staffing levels. Each of these factors can be influenced by the state and federal legislatures. It is important to recognize that each anesthesiologist and anesthesiologist in training can participate in the political process by meeting with their representatives, by writing letters to the editor, as well as by joining their state anesthesia PAC (Political Action Committee) as well as ASAPAC (American Society of Anesthesiologists Political Action Committee). Each state PAC sponsors an annual session where anesthesiologists can meet with their own legislators and present their viewpoint on pending legislation. It is important to recognize that nurse anesthetists are also lobbying for their views and their recent successes in gaining independent privileges is testimony to their determination to influence the political process.

As an example of political involvement, The New York State Society of Anesthesiologists sponsors a yearly trip to the state capital, Albany, to allow attending and resident staff to meet and educate their legislators. For several hours, the physicians fan out and meet with legislative staff as well as individual public officials. These meetings typically start with an introduction that educates the official about how one becomes an anesthesiologist and then moves onto one or two position points. It is important to focus on individual pieces of pending legislation that can have an outsized influence on anesthesia practice. Because many differing versions of bills are introduced, it is important to identify by bill number what will be helpful and what can be harmful to the profession. The legislators can then sign on as a sponsor or stand in opposition to it. The ASAPAC sponsors a similar event in the nation's capital. The goal at each event is to educate and convince legislators about the practice of anesthesia and how legislation is impacting this practice.

Another way to influence legislators is by holding fundraisers for their reelection. "Money is mother's milk for politicians" is an oft-heard expression, but holding a small fundraiser in honor of a local elected official will go a long way to gaining one-on-one access where the case can be made for a particular policy issue. The need to raise money for reelection is driven by the campaign cycle, and while some legislators are elected to 6-year terms (i.e., US Senators), others are in virtual constant campaign mode (i.e., US representatives). By contacting the legislative staff, dates that are available for fundraisers are readily obtained.

Charitable Giving

Lastly, anesthesiologists may participate directly in charitable giving. Various organizations, such as the World Federation of Societies of Anesthesiologists, coordinate projects to raise money and provide supplies and education to medical practitioners in disadvantaged areas of the world [12]. One of the most notable enterprises is Lifebox, organized by DR Enright, an anesthesiologist in Canada, initially to provide pulse oximeters to all operating rooms, worldwide. As she notes, "Our vision isn't just about distributing hardware and it doesn't stop with pulse oximetry. The provision of equipment is a nod, not a solution, to the dangerous shortfalls in global health provision. Education, training, and peer support are key. Lifebox is working for sustainable changes of practice that will ultimately raise the safety and quality standards of global healthcare." Through lectures and charitable events, DR Enright has raised millions of dollars.

Some organizations such as the New York State Society of Anesthesiologists have established 501c3 programs to help offset the cost of the international scholar program. Anesthesiologists may also contribute to nonmedical charitable causes, such as public welfare and arts organizations. While anesthesiology trainees may not have the financial means to make large monetary donations to these efforts, they are more than able to take roles in coordinating and administering such funds. Like medical mission work, this is an excellent way to gain a broader picture of the world's socioeconomic landscape, as well as a satisfying means of helping those less fortunate. In particular, participation in any charity related to healthcare can be a way to gain a greater perspective on and appreciation for the way inequalities can impact well-being and how these obstacles can be overcome.

Summary

While most of modern medicine still focuses on the individual patient-doctor interaction, this is not the only venue in which anesthesiologists are able to interact with the public. By broadening their interactions with patients and other nonmedical individuals through community outreach, trainees and practitioners develop flexibility, interpersonal skills, and the openness needed to handle whatever type of practice environment they may enter after graduation. In addition to the direct benefit outreach activities may have on anesthesiologists, patients, and other individuals, such pursuits can also lead to increased visibility and more positive public image for anesthesiology as a specialty. There seems to be a case where a little extra effort invested during residency can reap great benefits for all anesthesiologists, the specialty, and the world at large.

References

1. Klafta JM, Roizen MF. Current understanding of patients' attitudes towards and preparations for anesthesia: a review. Anesth Analg. 1996;83(6):1314–21.
2. Icahn School of Medicine at Mount Sinai. http://icahn.mssm.edu/departments-and-institutes/anesthesiology/about-us/history-of-the-mount-sinai-department-of-anesthesiology/community-service

3. ACGME Outcome Project. 2001. www.acgme.org/outcome
4. Roth R, Stensland K, Frost E. International surgical missions; More than just operate and leave. Association of University Anesthesiologists annual meeting, Miami, Poster presentation; 2013.
5. Soto RG, et al. Teaching systems-based competency in anesthesiology residency: development of an education and assessment tool. J Grad Med Educ. 2010;2(2):250–9.
6. Flores G. Language barriers to health care in the United States. N Engl J Med. 2006;355:229–31.
7. New York State Society of Anesthesiologists. www.nyssa-pga.org/members.aspx
8. Cassella C. Oxygen: a novel. New York: Simon and Schuster; 2009.
9. Pascoe W. Breathing for two: a life in anesthesiology. Washington, DC: Tinderbox; 2013.
10. Dhar P. Before the scalpel: what everyone should know about anesthesia. New Haven, CT: Tell Me Press; 2010.
11. Johna S, Rahman S. Humanity before science: narrative medicine, clinical practice, and medical education. Perm J. 2011;15(4):92–4.
12. World Society of Federations of Anesthesiologists. www.anaesthesiologists.org/about-us/charitable-donations

Chapter 18
Substance Abuse Recognition and Prevention Through Education

Ethan O. Bryson

Introduction

Despite ongoing research into the nature of addiction and a greater understanding of the factors which predispose some of our colleagues to this disease, the rate of substance abuse by anesthesia providers has remained constant over the last 40 years [1]. We have still not been able to reduce the number of anesthesia care personnel who become affected each year, making the promotion of educational videos and other materials that directly address the issue of substance abuse and anesthesia personnel even more important. The specter of addiction still remains a major issue in the anesthesia workplace, and each year 1–2 % of anesthesia care providers (ACPs) become addicted to the anesthetic agents they are tasked with administering to patients, leading some to ask: "Is addiction an occupational hazard for those involved in the practice of Anesthesiology?" Sadly death is the initial presentation in some 15 % of cases [2]. Because of the nature of anesthesia drugs, when they are self-administered, the risk for drug-related death is extremely high and the incidence of successful suicide attempts is greater than when other drugs are used. Implementing a program of education for individuals in training in anesthesiology which emphasizes early detection of afflicted colleagues and the unique risks inherent to the practice of anesthesia is essential and should be a regular part of every practice's wellness program.

E.O. Bryson, M.D. (✉)
Department of Anesthesiology and Psychiatry, The Icahn School of Medicine at Mount Sinai, 1 Gustave L Levy Plave, Box 1010, New York, NY, USA
e-mail: ethan.bryson@mountsinai.org

Background

In 1973 The American Medical Association (AMA) first formally recognized the problem of the impaired physician by publishing the "Sick Physician" Report, making public the notion that physicians are not immune to psychiatric disease, including substance abuse. The authors asserted that physicians have substantial issues with alcohol and drug abuse/dependence as well as other psychiatric illnesses and an increased risk for suicide [3]. They suggested that physicians have a responsibility to other physician colleagues as well as to their patients to address these issues and called for the establishment of diversion programs managed by state medical societies to identify and treat these people. In addition to identification and treatment, they called for the creation of programs aimed at prevention through education of medical students and residents.

At the time the notion that a physician might succumb to the problems of drug or alcohol addiction was altogether foreign. Physicians were seen as somehow "above the fray" and immune to these problems. Possibly because so much of what healthcare professionals do is not understood by the general public, this mystique of the healer as somehow different than the patient had persisted for generations. Physicians are often bright, strong-willed people. As a group they have faith in the ability of intellect and information to solve problems and effectively treat patients with medicines every day. The knowledge of drug actions and interactions can give healthcare professionals a false sense of control when they use these agents on themselves.

In the late 1980s, the American Association of Nurse Anesthetists (AANA), led by Diana Quinlan, formally recognized the significant risk for addiction in their membership with the creation of educational programs designed to provide a safety net for CRNAs who had become addicted to anesthetic agents. In a significant policy shift, their leadership began to advocate in favor of access to treatment for addicted certified registered nurse anesthetists (CRNAs) over punishment and licensure revocation for addicted ACPs. These efforts were sadly spurred on by the unfortunate overdose death of Jan Stewart, one of the former AANA Presidents, in the early 1990s, resulting in larger and wider efforts to educate members. Following the lead of their nursing colleagues, the physician members of The American Society of Anesthesiologists (ASA) formed a Committee on Occupational Health of Operating Room Personnel in 1990, headed at its inception by Dr. William Arnold. The resulting Task Force on Chemical Dependence was formed in an attempt to provide practical answers to the problem of drug addiction in anesthesia personnel. Bill Arnold and Diana Quinlan began the effort to educate all ACPs about the dangers of substance abuse which continues to this day.

Educators realized very quickly that media such as film and video could be effectively used to bring the very dramatic real-life stories of addiction, as told by the recovering addict and the family, friends, and colleagues of the addict who had overdosed, to a wide audience. Dr. Tom Hornbein, then Chairman of Anesthesia at the University of Washington, worked closely with Dr. John Lecky, a self-acknowledged recovering addict who later became a strong voice against substance abuse, to develop the first of the Wearing Masks series. Originally conceived and produced with the intention of reducing the frequency and devastating effects of the disease of addiction, the Wearing Masks series now consists of 11 video segments totaling over 3 h of material produced over a 13-year period.

Today the drive to educate the public about the dangers of the impaired healthcare professional has expanded to include all persons with access to highly addictive and dangerous prescription drugs. The book "Addicted Healers: 5 Key Signs Your Healthcare Professional May Be Drug Impaired" (September 2012, New Horizon Press) addresses the issue of the impaired healthcare professional through both the eyes of the medical professional and the eyes of the patient. It is written in nonmedical terms in an attempt to bring knowledge of this issue to a greater percentage of the population and encourage a call for action from the public. As our healthcare system continues to change, more and more of what healthcare professionals are expected to do will be market driven, including demands for substance abuse education and policy change.

Several hypotheses have been proposed to answer the question "What makes some people prone to addiction while others are not?" Some have suggested there is an association with a propensity towards addiction in persons who display novelty-seeking behavior traits, with persons identified as having fewer dopamine-inhibiting receptors being at higher risk. Some have pointed to what appears to be self-medication of symptoms associated with comorbid psychiatric disorders as a risk factor and cited the higher relapse risk in this group as evidence to support this theory. The proximity to large quantities of highly addictive drugs may put persons who are at risk but may not otherwise develop the disease in an environment which triggers a desire to self-administer. Still others suggest that chronic exposure is to blame, citing evidence that chronic opioid abuse leads to physical and chemical changes in the brain that directly increase drug craving. Regardless of why they start, the addict who continues to use drugs inappropriately does so not because of a conscious psychological choice but due to a physiological urge as a direct result of chemical changes within their brain [4].

How Common Is Substance Abuse in Anesthesia Care Providers?

As recently as 2007 it has been reported that between 10 and 15 % of all ACPs will abuse drugs or alcohol at some point in their career [5]. This reinforces the notion that these healthcare professionals (anesthesiologists at any stage of their training or practice and CRNAs) have the same propensity to develop the disease of addiction as any other member of the population. Medical or nursing students are members of the general population long before they matriculate so there is no reason to believe that they would have any less risk once they begin to practice as healthcare professionals. As many as 80 % of US anesthesiology residency programs have reported experience with impaired residents, and sadly 19 % of these programs reported at least one pretreatment fatality. A survey of controlled drug misuse by CRNAs conducted by Bell et al. in 1999 suggests that rates of addiction in the CRNA population are similar [6]. In the investigation conducted by Bell, researchers surveyed through anonymous query 2,500 practicing CRNAs and discovered that 9.8 % had misused controlled medications at some point within their career.

When we compare rates of impairment across medical specialties, addiction impacts anesthesiologists at rates similar to other medical professions. The total number of impaired professionals is similar from specialty to specialty, and this mirrors the larger population by region. What does stand out, however, is the increased incidence of addiction to specific types of drugs within this population and the higher risk of drug-related death among the anesthesia care professionals who abuse these drugs. The drugs that ACPs are more likely to abuse are the so-called "major" opioids, highly addictive agents such as fentanyl, sufentanil, and hydromorphone, but abuse of propofol, ketamine, midazolam, nitrous oxide, and the volatile anesthetics, basically anything that can be injected, snorted, inhaled, or swallowed, has been reported [7, 8]. These agents have a very narrow therapeutic index when self-administered, which explains why death from unintended overdose is often the presenting sign of addiction. The risk for death in this population is higher in the first 5 years after graduation and remains increased over that of other medical professionals [9].

It is difficult to estimate the actual number of anesthesia care professionals who will present with impairment related to drug or alcohol addiction each year, but the majority of investigations suggest that close to 1.0 % of faculty members practicing for more than 5 years, 1.5 % of residents and junior faculty, and 1–2 % of CRNAs will become addicted each year [10]. These numbers represent only the known cases, that is, those that come to the attention of authorities because of overdose, witnessed self-injection, drug- or alcohol-related arrests, or referral to treatment programs. The actual number of ACPs diverting anesthetics for personal use may be much higher, as many affected individuals may enter treatment without coming to the attention of the authorities or the medical board.

Denial and the Identification of the Impaired Healthcare Professional

The addict does not often recognize that he or she has a problem, and as a result, treatment is seldom spontaneously sought. Because of this, denial can present a major obstacle to both the identification and the treatment of the addict, especially the addicted healthcare professional. It is especially important to recognize that denial is not limited to the addict. Often the colleagues of an addicted healthcare professional do not recognize behavior that in retrospect is obviously related to addiction.

There are behavior patterns which may suggest a colleague might have a substance abuse problem, and all anesthesia personnel should be aware of what to look for.

Identifying the substance-abusing ACP is often difficult as the addicted ACP may appear quite functional until very late in the course of the disease. These addicts need to remain close to their supply of drugs, so they may remain extraordinarily attentive at work, while leaving all other aspects of their life unattended to. Changes in behavior such as periods of irritability, anger, euphoria, and depression are frequently noted. The addict will begin to withdraw from family, friends, and leisure activities in favor of spending more time at the hospital, even when off duty, often volunteering for extra call.

Some of the changes typically observed in the addicted ACP include the following:

- Withdrawal from family, friends, and leisure activities as more time is spent at work where the drug can be used
- Mood swings, with periods of depression or bad moods alternating with periods of euphoria or gregariousness, depending upon whether the addicted provider is high or in withdrawal
- Increasing episodes of anger, irritability, and hostility and increased sensitivity to criticism
- Spending more time at the hospital, even when off duty, often with odd intentions (coming in on a Saturday afternoon to "set up" a room for a case scheduled for late on Monday) in order to obtain and use drugs
- Volunteering for extra call as an excuse to remain at work, offering to "set up" rooms for other providers
- Refusing relief for lunch or coffee breaks, so that their diversion of drugs for personal use is not discovered
- Requesting frequent bathroom breaks, during which the addicted provider frequently self-administers drugs
- Failure to respond to pager, difficult to arouse when on night call
- Signing out increasing amounts of narcotics or quantities inappropriate for the given case so that more is available for self-administration
- Frequent "ampoule breakage" and increased "waste"
- Weight loss and pale skin, as less time and energy are spent taking care of themselves
- Wearing long sleeves or other clothing designed to hide physical evidence of self-injection

By the time the user realizes he or she has become addicted, it is often too late to quit without treatment. How long this take depends on the drug. For example, it may take years for an alcoholic to deteriorate to the point where abuse becomes apparent, but it may only take a few months for a fentanyl addiction to become apparent. One of the reasons an addiction to one of the major opioids becomes apparent so much more quickly is tolerance to the effects of these medications. For drugs with a short half-life, tolerance can develop rapidly. Addicts have reported self-administration of 1,000 μg of fentanyl in a single injection just to relieve the symptoms of withdrawal. For the ACP addicted to these drugs, the need for increasing amounts of opioids soon drives diversion behavior which can ultimately harm patients.

Diversion

So powerful is the disease of addiction and the need for the drug that otherwise reasonable and intelligent people will resort to seemingly incredulous behavior in order to obtain their drug of choice. When the need to obtain and use the drug is the addicts' foremost priority, any oath sworn long ago to "do no harm" is tossed by the wayside. Addicts have reported charting that they administered their drug of choice to a patient when in fact the patient received either saline or nothing at all. In order to cover up the effects of surgery with inadequate or no pain medications, the addict may use inhalational agents and beta-blockers. Some addicted ACPs have reported to substitute a syringe of saline or esmolol for their opioid of choice while giving a relief break to one of their colleagues or even rummaging through sharp containers looking for small amounts of discarded opioids.

Addicts quickly become proficient at removing controlled substances from secure places. Automated dispensing machines do not prevent diversion. Often the security features of these machines can be defeated, and at best they only keep a record of who was logged in when the drugs were removed. Drugs may be removed from glass ampoules and replaced with another liquid without evidence of tampering.

The following cases represent ACPs who are at different points in their disease of addiction. Though it may not be obvious from their behavior at the time, they were each subsequently found to be diverting opioids for personal use. Without definitive proof it can be easy to dismiss their behavior as either "appropriate under the circumstances" or "an anomaly" and not representative drug-seeking behavior. If you find yourself making excuses for them, remember that denial is not limited to the addict.

Case 1

John is an anesthesia resident in his second year of training. He seemed a little more nervous than the rest of his classmates when he started residency but it seems that he has now settled into a routine. He likes to have a few drinks after call and usually heads over to Hanratty's with whoever will go with him before going home in the morning. Last week he "got into it" with one of the more demanding surgeons during a particularly stressful case and his attending had to be called into the room to straighten things out.

Because there exists a considerable association between chemical dependence and other psychopathology, John's behavior needs to be put into context. It is possible that he may have an underlying anxiety disorder or other psychiatric issue, but these cannot be diagnosed until he has been free of drug and alcohol abuse for a period of months. Polysubstance abuse is common, and addicts often substitute one drug for another if they cannot obtain their drug of choice. As it turns out, John has recently started drinking heavily when he is away from the hospital because he does not have access to the opioids he has become addicted to. In many cases, binge or heavy drinking during residency predates the discovery that the resident has been abusing other drugs as well.

Case 2

Sara is a recent graduate of a top-notch nurse anesthesia program. Despite her successful completion of CRNA school and her new job, she isn't quite sure she has made the right decision about a career in anesthesiology. Sara often complains about behaviors or circumstances that others find normal but that she believes are personally directed at her. She seems distracted by her upcoming wedding and spends a lot of time either on the phone or surfing the web during cases. She asks for frequent "bathroom" breaks and is often gone for longer than she should be. She is either irritable or distracted and shows little interest in work.

Mood swings are not uncommon in the addict but some people are just "moody" so it can be difficult to tell if this is a sign of addiction or not. Changes in behavior are more telling, and the person who used to have an easy-going personality but now becomes irritated at small and unimportant things usually has something else going on. The substitution of a drug for a significant other can lead to relationship difficulties and infidelity is common. In this case Sara began using opioids very early on during her training and has now become apathetic to everything else.

Case 3

Brian is a junior staff attending. He is well respected and liked by his peers. He hardly ever complains about having to stay late and is known as a "team player," often volunteering for extra call or refusing relief at the end of the day. Lately he looks a little more "run down" than usual, but that can easily be explained by the long hours he has been working.

Behaviors such as this may make the addict appear to be quite functional. Many new members of the attending staff pick up extra calls or volunteer for the tougher cases to either make a little extra money or to make a name for themselves in the group. It can be difficult to accept that a problem in a colleague is a result of addiction, but remember that your failure to initiate an investigation because of "uncertainty" masked as concern for the individual is denial.

Case 4

Jan is a senior resident and is on her first cardiac rotation. She says she is enjoying it but she looks exhausted. She has been working late every night this week because

Table 18.1 Signs and symptoms typically observed in the addicted anesthesia provider experiencing opioid withdrawal

- Irritability
- Dysphoria
- Intense drug craving
- Nausea and vomiting
- Diarrhea
- Anorexia
- Muscle aches and or back pain
- Lacrimation
- Rhinorrhea
- Diaphoresis
- Mydriasis
- Yawning
- Fever
- Insomnia
- Amenorrhea

one of the cardiac fellows is out sick, but she was relieved early today and told to go home. Instead she goes to the control desk and offers to work an extra paid call, admitting she's tired but that she could really use the extra money.

The opioid addict who is in acute withdrawal is desperate. Jan is displaying some of the classic physical signs of acute opioid withdrawal: pale, cool, clammy skin, and constant sniffling. Other signs and symptoms are listed in Table 18.1. Despite your justifiable concern, do not confront the individual yourself. Addicts have been known to commit suicide once they have been discovered as they realize that the world as they know it is about to change forever. In this situation immediately contact a member of your departments' wellness committee who will arrange for an intervention to take place. Make sure the individual remains supervised and in a safe place, without tipping them off that they have been discovered. An intervention needs to take place and should be handled by trained individuals.

Intervention

A member of the department's wellness committee should be familiar with the intervention protocol. It is essential that a trained interventionist be present at all times. When assembling the group for the intervention, one must be sensitive to gender. A group comprised entirely of males on the intervention team is inappropriate if the individual is a female. A larger group is usually better than a smaller one. The individual's spouse, family members, friends, and colleagues should be included if possible, indeed anyone who is close with the individual so long as they are supportive of the intervention and will not be disruptive. All the evidence which supports diversion and inappropriate drug use, including a properly collected drug screen, should be available. Urination must be witnessed, chain of custody protocol must be maintained, and specimen should be split for secondary verification. The person should never be allowed to leave the intervention alone and should not be permitted to drive under any circumstances. Impaired individuals may become suicidal once the gravity of the situation they are in becomes apparent and they may have a "stash" in their car or locker. It is important to make arrangements for direct transfer to an inpatient facility prior to the intervention.

Addicts should not decide their treatment; they are sick and they will minimize the problem. As last resort, if the addict is adamant that they do not have a problem, suggesting that the matter should be turned over to the police or the drug enforcement agency may cause them to finally admit that they have a serious problem.

What Happens After the Intervention?

Once a referral is made to an inpatient facility that specializes in the treatment of healthcare professionals, admission should occur as soon as a ready bed is available. If given time, there is a very real possibility that the addict will change his/her mind about entering treatment. It is important to arrange for treatment in a facility with a healthcare professional program so the affected individual can develop the support of other similarly affected HCPs [11]. There are currently no programs in the United States that admit only HCPs, but there are several that offer programs for HCPs within the larger inpatient population. Talbott in Florida, Marworth in Pennsylvania, and Hazelden in Minnesota are examples of these types of facilities. ACPs represent a special case within the group of HCPs as a whole. Because of the nature of the drugs to which they typically become addicted, ACPs are sent for residential treatment that may last from 2 months to a year or more.

The intensive inpatient treatment model involves staff contact extending up to 12 h per day, 7 days per week. In this environment the addicted ACP is removed from the stresses of daily life as well as from access to alcohol and drugs. Participation in self-help groups is a vital component in the therapy and essential for sustained recovery once the addict is discharged to either a halfway house or directly to the community.

The successful recovery program will include elements of all of the following:

- Detoxification
- Monitored abstinence
- Education
- Exposure to self-help groups
- Psychotherapy

Can the ACP in Recovery Return to Work?

Most states allow ACPs, both physicians and CRNAs, to return to work so long as they do so while under the supervision of a physician or nursing health and well-being organization such as those that are sponsored by the state medical or nursing society. The required monitoring contracts are usually a minimum of 5 years in length and stipulate that the individual must maintain regular contact with the caseworker and submit to worksite observation or supervision as well as to random urine drug and alcohol screens. The chances that the ACP who is compliant with these stipulations will not relapse are good, provided he/she remains in a program of complete abstinence from all mood-altering drugs. Facilitated group psychotherapy with other recovering healthcare professionals is an important part of early recovery and is usually mandated for a period of 2–3 years or longer for individuals who wish to return to clinical practice. Regular attendance and participation in self-help fellowships such as AA or NA increases the likelihood of success and is encouraged if not also mandated. Monitoring contracts have been shown to increase physician recovery rate by 20–30 % as compared to physician controls [12].

Physicians and nurses are typically highly motivated to complete programs and continue to practice medicine or nursing, but whether ACPs in recovery should be allowed to return to the operating room remains highly controversial. Even though participants who remain compliant with their prescribed program and are able to remain abstinent at 5-year follow-up [13], many have pointed out that when a member of this group does relapse, often the presenting sign is death. Most states have a policy of making a decision regarding return to work on a case-by-case basis, regardless of the level of training or years of experience.

The Risk for Relapse

Despite the substantial success rates at 5-year follow-up for healthcare professionals compliant with a mandated program of recovery, it should be remembered that addiction is a chronic disease and relapse is expected. The key is to be able to identify behaviors which suggest that a relapse is imminent before the addict actually picks up the drug. Often the addict in recovery is the first person to recognize these behaviors for what they are, which is why maintaining active involvement in the recovery community is so important. Individuals who have undergone treatment are still at risk for relapse, even several years or even decades after their last use [14].

Factors which are associated with an increased risk of relapse include:

- A family history of substance use disorder
- The use of a major opioid
- The presence of a coexisting psychiatric disorder
- Nonparticipation in a monitoring program

Strategies to Prevent Diversion and Substance Abuse

Random Drug Screening

For some reason random drug screening in the medical profession remains a contentious issue. Random drug testing has been shown to demonstrate a positive deterrent effect in every branch of the US military as well as the Department of Transportation

(DOT), Federal Transit Administration (FTA), Federal Aviation Administration (FAA), and Federal Railroad Administration (FRA). A strict no-tolerance drug policy coupled with random urine testing increases safety in the workplace as evidenced by a statistically significant decline in the number of reportable accidents after the implementation of such a policy. Despite its proven efficacy, very few nonmilitary programs actually have true random drug screening. Many hospitals have preemployment or for-cause drug screens. Perhaps it would be prudent to implement a program of random testing of anesthesia providers.

For random drug screening to be effective, the Substance Abuse and Mental Health Services Administration (SAMHSA) guidelines must be followed. Specimen collection must be truly random and not predictable and micturition must be witnessed. If costs are a concern or to avoid singling out individual members of the department, some programs collect a specimen from everybody in the department and then randomly select which samples to actually test. When the sample is collected, each specimen should be split. Half of the sample is tested initially and half is frozen in case there is a discrepancy or a contested positive result [15]. Drug testing is then conducted via radioimmunoassay (RIA) which is sensitive but not specific. RIA is the screening test used to rule *out* drug use and any positive result must then be confirmed with gas chromatography/mass spectrometry (GC/MS). GC/MS is the confirmatory test used to rule *in* drug use. Since most standard substance abuse assays do not include the drugs typically abused by ACPs, a specific request must be made to include fentanyl, propofol, ketamine, or other such agents.

Monitoring Use Patterns

As the number of hospitals employing anesthesia information management systems (AIMS) increases, it is becoming easier to evaluate for use patterns suspicious for diversion. ACPs whose use of opioids or level of controlled substance wastage is greater than two standard deviations above the mean for the group can be flagged for further evaluation. Automated dispenser transactions can be examined to identify transactions which occur on canceled cases, after case completion or even in a different location.

How Should Waste Drugs Be Handled?

Since most drugs appear the same to the naked eye, the answer to the question "What's actually in that syringe?" could be just about anything. In the case of the addicted ACP, it's most likely saline. All waste drugs should be returned to the pharmacy and assayed by handheld refractometer to determine that the liquid matches the expected characteristics of the drug indicated on the label. Any questionable samples should be sent out for further analysis.

Conclusion

As more and more emphasis is placed on cost containment and increased productivity, healthcare professionals of all ilk are constantly being asked to work harder, for longer hours, and frequently for less pay. In this environment it is crucial that we not overlook the importance of taking time to educate people on the topic of addiction. The actual cost to a physician group or hospital that results from the damage caused by an addicted healthcare professional is difficult to quantify, but estimates range from $450,000 to $600,000 for expenses related to the death of an employee from a diversion-related overdose alone. If patient harm has occurred and litigation for damages is involved, the cost increases dramatically. In addition to the financial costs associated with such an event, there is the stigma and negative publicity that ultimately results from media coverage of the incident. There exists a significant risk for damage to the specific institution and harm to the profession as a whole. It would seem expedient and short sighted not to invest the time and resources required to put in place an effective program of education aimed at increasing addiction awareness in each workplace.

For an educational campaign to be effective, it must not only inform but also provide a suitable safety net for those at risk and encourage the well-being of healthcare professionals at every level in an organization. These programs need to be targeted to students, SRNAs, residents as new physicians with possibly immature coping skills, newly graduated physicians and CRNAs, and senior-level members of the department or private practice group as all members of the anesthesia care team at every level of training and experience are at risk for developing addiction.

References

1. Bryson EO, Silverstein JH. Addiction and substance abuse in anesthesiology. Anesthesiology. 2008;109(5):905–17.
2. Collins GB, McAllister MS, Jensen M, Gooden TA. Chemical dependency treatment outcomes of residents in anesthesiology: results of a survey. Anesth Analg. 2005;101:1457–62.
3. AMA Council on Mental Health. The sick physician: impairment by psychiatric disorders, including alcoholism and drug dependence. JAMA. 1973;223:684–7.
4. Malison RT, Best SE, Wallace EA, McCance E, Laruelle M, Zoghbi SS, Baldwin RM, Seibyl JS, Hoffer PB, Price LH. Euphorigenic doses of cocaine reduce [123I]beta-CIT SPECT measures of dopamine transporter availability in human cocaine addicts. Psychopharmacology (Berl). 1995;122:358–62.
5. Baldisseri MR. Impaired healthcare professional. Crit Care Med. 2007;35(2):S106–16.
6. Bell DM, McDonough JP, Ellison JS, Fitzhugh EC. Controlled drug misuse by Certified Registered Nurse Anesthetists. AANA J. 1999;67(2):133–40.
7. Kintz P, Villain M, Dumestre V, Cirimele V. Evidence of addiction by anesthesiologists as documented by hair analysis. Forensic Sci Int. 2005;153:81–4.
8. Wischmeyer PE, Johnson BR, Wilson JE, Dingmann C, Bachman HM, Roller E, Tran ZV, Henthorn TK. A survey of propofol abuse in academic anesthesia programs. Anesth Analg. 2007;105:1066–71.

9. Alexander BH, Checkoway H, Nagahama SI, Domino KB. Cause-specific mortality risks of anesthesiologists. Anesthesiology. 2000;93:922–30.
10. Booth JV, Grossman D, Moore J, Lineberger C, Reynolds JD, Reves JG, Sheffield D. Substance abuse among physicians: a survey of academic anesthesiology programs. Anesth Analg. 2002;95:1024–30.
11. Hankes L, Bissell L. Health professionals. In: Lowinson JH, Ruiz P, Millman RB, editors. Substance abuse: a comprehensive textbook. Baltimore: Williams and Wilkins; 1992. p. 897–908.
12. Shore JH. The Oregon experience with impaired physicians on probation, an eight-year follow-up. JAMA. 1987;257:2931–4.
13. Skipper GE. Anesthesiologists with substance use disorders: a 5-year outcome study from 16 state physician health programs. Anesth Analg. 2009;109(3):891–6.
14. Domino KB, Hornbein TF, Polissar NF, Renner G, Johnson J, Alberti S, Hankes L. Risk factors for relapse in health care professionals with substance use disorders. JAMA. 2005;293:1453–60.
15. Bryson EO, Hamza H. The drug seeking anesthesia provider. Int Anesthesiol Clin. 2011;49(1):157–71.

Index

A
AAMC. *See* Association of American Medical Colleges (AAMC)
ABA. *See* American Board of Anesthesiology (ABA)
Accreditation Council for Continuing Medical Education (ACCME), 174, 176, 182
Accreditation Council for Graduate Medical Education (ACGME), 120
  application process, 42
  duty hours, 51–53
  fellowships, 66–67
  institutional requirements, 42–43
Aeginata, Paulus, 2
AMA. *See* American Medical Association (AMA)
AMA Physician's Recognition Award (AMA PRA), 176
AMA PRA Category 1 Credit™, 176, 181
American Association of Nurse Anesthetists (AANA), 230
American Board of Anesthesiology (ABA), 207
  candidate status policy, 108
  examination development, 100–101
  ITE, 102–103, 114–116
  LLSA program, 118–120
  Maintenance of Certification, 111–112
  Part 1 (written) examination, 103–104
  Part 2 (oral) examination
    Blueprint, 105
    Deficient Attributes, 106, 107
    external psychometric firm, 106
    four-point rating scale, 106–107
    many-facet Rasch model, 107
    35-min exam session, 105
    4-point Likert scale, 106
    preoperative information, 106
    qualities and attributes, 105
    standardized guided questions, 105
  staged examination system
    ADVANCED Exam, 109
    APPLIED Examination, 110
    BASIC Exam, 108–109
  subspecialty certification, 110–111
  test security, 113
American Board of Internal Medicine (ABIM), 167, 168
American Board of Medical Specialties (ABMS), 108, 111, 117–118, 180
American Journal of Surgery, 9
American Medical Association (AMA), 174, 178, 230
American Society of Anesthesiologists, 8–10
Anesthesia
  history
    education and medical schools, 9–10
    entertainment, 2–3
    fatalities, 5
    idiosyncratic death, 4
    in nineteenth century, 3–4
    response rate, 5–6
    "soporific sponge," 2
    textbooks, 7
    in twentieth century, 11
    in twenty-first century, 11
  mentorship (*see* Mentorship)
  operating room (*see* Operating room (OR))
Anesthesia care providers (ACPs), 231–234, 237–238
Anesthesia Knowledge Test (AKT), 50, 141

Anesthesiology residents, 142–143.
    See also Residency training
    assessment
        accountability, 135
        audit technique, 136
        of competence, 135
        comprehensiveness, 134
        direct observation, 136–137
        vs. evaluation, 131, 133–134
        feasibility, 134–135
        flexibility, 135
        formative assessment, 131, 133
        mentorship, 137
        oral examination, 138
        OSCE, 137
        peer review, 138
        portfolio assessment, 138–139
        reliability, 134
        self-assessment, 139–140
        simulation, 140
        standardized patients, 140–141
        summative assessment, 131, 133
        validity, 134
        written examination, 141
    Likert scales, 130, 142
    NAS, 141–142
Anesthesiology training, 183–184, 192
ASA Continuing Education (ACE) program, 119, 125, 179
Association of American Medical Colleges (AAMC), 196, 200
Association of Anaesthetists of Great Britain and Ireland (AAGBI), 207

B
Bernard, Claude, 4
Board certification. *See* American Board of Anesthesiology (ABA)
Buchanan, T.D., 8

C
Canadian Anesthesiologists' Society International Education Foundation (CAS IEF), 207
Cardiothoracic anesthesiology, 62–63
CCM. *See* Critical care medicine (CCM)
Certified registered nurse anesthetists (CRNAs), 230–232
Classroom teaching
    audience, 23–25
    slides and materials, 24
Clinical anesthesia, year 1 (CA-1), 142

Clinical anesthesia, year 2 (CA-2), 142
Clinical anesthesia, year 3 (CA-3), 142
Clinical base year (CBY), 48–49
CME. *See* Continuing medical education (CME)
Communication skills, 77–78
Community outreach
    charity, 226–227
    electronic, print, and blogs, 225
    free care and access to care, 217–220
    international scholar programs, 220
    medical missions, 217–220
    observerships, 220
    opportunities, 216–217
    political process, 226
    systems-based practice
        definition, 221
        public education, 221–225
Continuing medical education (CME), 118–120
    accreditation criteria, 174–175
    AMA PRA, 176
    CME activities
        licensure, credentialing, and privileging, 180
        lifelong learning, 179–180
        MOCA, 180–181
    definition, 173
    funding, 182
    origin, 174
    presentation formats
        enduring materials, 177
        Internet point-of-care learning, 178–179
        journal-based, 177
        live activities, 176–177
        manuscript review for journals, 178
        PI CME, 178
        test item writing, 177
Critical care medicine (CCM), 60–61
Critical incidents reporting (CIR), 28
Culturally Centered Mentorship Model (CCMM), 90

D
Debriefing Assessment for Simulation in Healthcare (DASH), 166

E
Educational research, 195, 202
    academic medical centers, 196
    conceptual frameworks, 196, 201

Index

data collection
    qualitative research, 198
    quantitative research, 198
    reliability, 199
    validity, 199
FAER, 202
IRB approval, 201
MedEdPORTAL Publications, 200
prospective study, 198
research question, 197
retrospective study, 197–198
Evidence-based medicine (EBM), 46

F
Faculty Mentoring Leadership Program, 96
Feedback
    retaliation, 151
    to superiors (*see* Superiors, feedback)
    teaching, 83
Fellowships
    ACGME, 66–67
    anesthesiology training, 59
    cardiothoracic anesthesiology, 62–63
    critical care medicine, 60–61
    non-accredited fellowships
        neurosurgical anesthesiology, 65
        obstetric anesthesiology, 64
        organ transplantation, 65
        regional anesthesiology, 65
    pain medicine, 61–62
    pediatric anesthesiology, 63–64
Foundation for Anesthesia Education and Research (FAER), 202

G
Gas chromatography/mass spectrometry (GC/MS), 239
General and Local Anesthetics, 7
Global health education
    definition, 206
    global health electives
        benefits of, 207–208
        challenges to, 209–210
        and departments, 209
    goals of, 206–207
    host departments and faculty, 210–211
    pre-mission preparation, 208–209
    role of ethics, 212
Graduate medical education (GME), 130
    ACGME general competencies, 131–133
    feedback to superiors (*see* Superiors, feedback)
    implications for, 131
    primary care programs, 138
Group of Anaesthetists in Training (GAT), 207

H
Hauer, Erich, 1
Honduran hospital, 217–219

I
International Association of Medical Science Educators (IAMSE), 200
International scholar programs, 220
Interprofessional education, 188
    definition, 185
    patient outcomes/service delivery, 189
In-training examination (ITE), 102–103, 114–116

L
Lifelong learning and self-assessment (LLSA), 118–120
Long Island Society of Anesthetists, 8–9
Louisiana State Health Sciences Center, 168

M
Maintenance of Certification (MOC), 111–112, 180
Maintenance of Certification in Anesthesiology (MOCA)
    ABA certification, expiration of, 124
    benefits of, 125–126
    components
        cognitive examination, 120, 181
        lifelong learning and self-assessment, 118–120, 181
        PPAI, 120–122
        professional standing assessment, 118, 180
    cost of, 124–125
    diplomates, 123
    evolution of, 126
    MOCA reporting, 123–124
    for non-time-limited certificate holder, 122
    for subspecialties, 122
Maintenance of Certification in Anesthesiology for Subspecialties (MOCA-SUBS) program, 100, 112–113, 122

Medical education
  CME (see Continuing medical education (CME))
  feedback to superiors, 148–149
    cultural aspects, 152–153
    message threat, effect of, 150–152
    recipient, receptivity of, 150–152
  GME (see Graduate medical education (GME))
  research in (see Educational research)
  SBME (see Simulation-based medical education (SBME))
Medical Simulation Corporation's SimSuite® technology, 168
Mentorship
  background, 87–88
  barriers, 95
  baseline survey, 92
  business models, 92
  career advancement, 92
  careers, effects of, 89
  CCMM, 90
  clinical setting, 89
  vs. coach, 88
  definition, 88
  ethnic minority faculty members, 89
  faculty evaluation, 94–95
  Faculty Mentoring Leadership Program, 96
  goals set, 92
  mentee/mentor assignments, 92
  mentorship program, 95–96
  middle-base/B-player, 91
  profile questionnaire, 92–93
  project development and grant submissions, 92
  publication process, 89
  role of, 88
  self-assessment surveys, 97
  types, 88
MOCA. See Maintenance of Certification in Anesthesiology (MOCA)
Multidisciplinary education
  awareness, 187
  complimentary, 188
  consultation, 187
  correlation, 188
  definition, 185
  history, 185–186
  interprofessional education, 188
  isolation, 187
  lack of support, 190
  "learning together," 188
  multiprofessional education, 188
  nesting, 188
  organization and implementation, 190
  palliative medicine, 191
  patient safety, 184
  "product champions," 189
  shared teaching, 188
  temporal coordination, 188
  three-dimensional approach, 186
  "transition driver," 190
  transprofessional education, 188
  "working together," 188
Multiple choice questions (MCQ), 104, 109, 120, 135, 141

N
Neurosurgical anesthesiology, 65
New York State (NYS) Fair, 222–224
New York State Society of Anesthesiologists (NYSSA), 222–224
Next Accreditation System (NAS), 141–142

O
Objective structured clinical examination (OSCE), 134, 135, 137
Observerships, 220
Obstetric anesthesiology, 64
Operating room (OR)
  communication barriers, 22–23
  emotional content, 20–21
  junior residents, 22
  learning environment, 18–19
  real-life experiences, 19–20
  root cause analysis
    action plan, 33
    active errors, 32
    chronological event sequence, 31
    latent errors, 32
    preventive measures, 33
  teaching, 73
  teaching schedule, 17–18
OR. See Operating room (OR)
Oral examination
  ABA board certification
    Blueprint, 105
    Deficient Attributes, 106, 107
    external psychometric firm, 106
    four-point rating scale, 106–107
    many-facet Rasch model, 107
    35-min exam session, 105
    4-point Likert scale, 106
    preoperative information, 106
    qualities and attributes, 105
    standardized guided questions, 105
  anesthesiology resident, 138
Organ transplantation, 65

Index

P
Pain medicine, 61–62
Pediatric anesthesiology, 63–64
Performance improvement (PI), 178
Practice performance assessment and improvement (PPAI), 119–121
 attestation process, 121–122
 case evaluation, 121
 simulation education course, 121
Problem-based learning (PBL), 81
Problem-based learning initiative (PBLI), 136
Professionalism, 77–78
Public education, 221–225

R
Radioimmunoassay (RIA), 239
Random drug screening, 238–239
RCA. *See* Root cause analysis (RCA)
Regional anesthesiology, 65
Reporter, interpreter, manager, educator (RIME), 135
Residency Review Committee (RRC), 131
Residency training
 ACGME, 42–43
 clinical-based milestones, 49
 clinical base year, 48–49
 clinical duties, 53
 educational program components
  EBM, 46
  good interpersonal and communication skills, 47
  minimum case requirements, 45
  patient care, 44
  PDSA cycle, 46
  professionalism, 47
  required didactic topics, 45
  systems-based practice, 47
 goals and objectives, 53
 history of, 41–42
 program personnel and appointments, 43–44
 research principle, 53
Root cause analysis (RCA)
 contributory factors, 29
 extubation failure
  action plan, 38
  active errors, 35, 37
  chronological event sequence, 35
  in-depth analysis, 35
  latent errors, 37
  preventive measures, 37–38
  production pressure, 37
 fire, in operating room
  action plan, 33
  active errors, 32
  chronological event sequence, 31
  latent errors, 32
  preventive measures, 33
 ideal and actual process flows, 29
Rovenstine, Emery, 10
Royal College of Anaesthetists (RCoA), 207

S
SBME. *See* Simulation-based medical education (SBME)
Self-Education and Evaluation. (SEE) program, 119
Simulation, 81–82
 application of, 166–168
 business awareness, 160
 certification, 167–168
 clinical skills, 163–164
 considerations and outcomes-based education, 168–169
 curriculum design, 161–163
 definition, 160
 integration of training simulations, 161, 162
 interactive experiences, 160
 problem solving, 160
 SBME (*see* Simulation-based medical education (SBME))
 team approach, simulated learning
  debriefing, 165–166
  facilitator, 165
  participants, 164–165
 team coordination, 160
 time management and organization, 160
Simulation-based medical education (SBME), 161
 clinical skills, 164
 deliberate practice, 163
 goals of, 167
 MOCA, 167
 team-oriented approach, 164
 translational science research, 169
Simulation-based team training (SBTT), 164
Simulation teaching, 81–82
Slides, 24
Standardized patients (SP), 137
Stanford University, 216
Substance abuse
 in ACPs, 231–232
  acute opioid withdrawal, 236
  anxiety disorder/psychiatric issue, 234
  cardiac rotation, 235
  frequent bathroom breaks, 235
  mood swings, 235
  polysubstance abuse, 234–235

Substance abuse (*cont.*)
    in recovery, 237–238
    signs and symptoms, 236
    volunteering for extra call/refusing relief, 235
  impaired healthcare professional, 232–233
  intervention, 236–237
  risk for relapse, 238
  strategies to
    monitoring use patterns, 239
    random drug screening, 238–239
    waste drugs, 239
Substance Abuse and Mental Health Services Administration (SAMHSA) guidelines, 239
Superiors, feedback
  anesthesiology, 149
  business and management sectors, 147–148
  medical education, 148–149
    cultural aspects, 152–153
    message threat, effect of, 150–152
    recipient, receptivity of, 150–152
  relationship filter, 155–156
  skills, 156
  strategies
    for residents, 154–155
    for teachers, 153
  UMMSM, 149–150

T
Targeted areas for improvement (TAFI), 131, 133
Teaching
  "active observation," 75–76
  anesthesiology clerkship, 70, 72–73
  classroom teaching
    audience, 23–25
    slides and materials, 24
  clinical exposure, 74
  clinical teacher, role of, 74–75
  communication skills and professionalism, 77–78
  conventional learning, 73
  domains, 71
  evaluation and feedback, 83
  fun and games, 82
  medical missions, 83
  medical student, role of, 73–74
  operating room, 73
  practice, scope of, 71–72
  problem-based learning, 81
  questioning, 75
  resident work hour restrictions, 71
  simulation teaching (*see* Simulation)
  stakeholder characteristics, 70
  team-based learning, 79–80
  technical skills, 76–77
  technology tools, 82–83
  time constraints, 74
  topic discussions, 80–81
  traditional lecture, 78–79
Team-based learning (TBL), 79–80

U
United States Medical Licensing Examinations (USMLE), 133
University of Miami Miller School of Medicine (UMMSM), 149–150, 156
University of Washington School of Medicine, 191

V
Vanderbilt University, 216

W
Working Group on Ethics Guidelines for Global Health Training (WEIGHT), 212
World Federation of Societies of Anaesthesiologists (WFSA), 211
World Health Organization (WHO), 61, 185
Written examination
  ABA board certification, 103–104
  anesthesiology resident, 141

The manufacturer's authorised representative in the EU is Springer Nature Customer Service Centre GmbH, Europaplatz 3, 69115 Heidelberg, Germany. If you have any concerns regarding our products, please contact ProductSafety@springernature.com

Printed and bound by CPI Group (UK) Ltd, Croydon, CR0 4YY

23/03/2026

02076446-0008